T0248054

All You Need is Rhythm & Grit

ALL YOU NEED IS RHYTHM & GRIT

Pegasus Books, Ltd.
148 West 37th Street, 13th Floor
New York, NY 10018

Copyright © 2024 by Cory Wharton-Malcolm

First Pegasus Books cloth edition May 2024

Book design by Heather Ryerson

Illustrations © Alice Mollon, 2024

All rights reserved. No part of this book may be reproduced in whole or in part without written permission from the publisher, except by reviewers who may quote brief excerpts in connection with a review in a newspaper, magazine, or electronic publication; nor may any part of this book be reproduced, stored in a retrieval system, or transmitted in any form or by any means electronic, mechanical, photocopying, recording, or other, without written permission from the publisher.

ISBN: 978-1-63936-660-6

10 9 8 7 6 5 4 3 2 1

Printed in the United States of America
Distributed by Simon & Schuster
www.pegasusbooks.com

All You Need is Rhythm & Grit

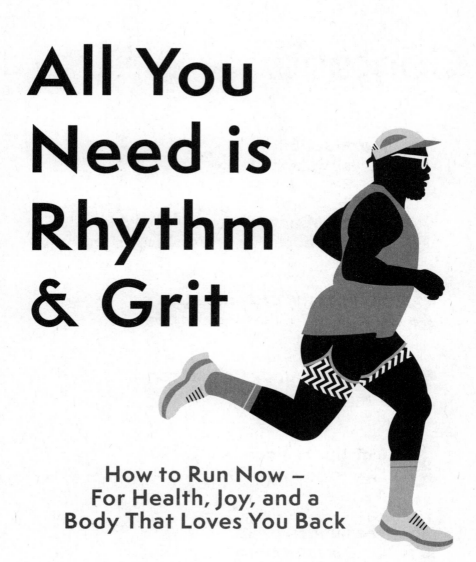

How to Run Now –
For Health, Joy, and a
Body That Loves You Back

Cory Wharton-Malcolm

PEGASUS BOOKS
NEW YORK LONDON

Contents

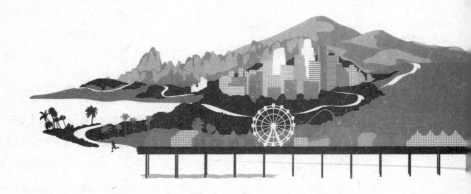

Do *you* *want* to run?

My name is Cory Wharton-Malcolm and I have been on this beautiful planet for a little over 40 years. I was born in London in St Thomas's Hospital overlooking the Thames, and though I have travelled a lot and lived elsewhere the gritty city of London has always been the place I call home.

Now I ask you, do you want to run? I mean, has the thought ever crossed your mind? Perhaps, for whatever reason, you've not yet found that thing that gets you out there. The motivation? The hook? The right vibe? People? Or energy? Something to pull you in?

Do you look at people running and think that that running thing looks great and you'd love to run like that . . . gracefully floating through the air, with a big grin on your face looking like you've not got a care in the world? But for some strange reason your mind wanders elsewhere and you begin to feel like that's a THEM thing, not a YOU thing? I've been there . . . But . . . What if I told you running *is* a YOU thing? What if I told you the only thing separating you and a run is YOU and that magical FIRST STEP? You may not aspire to run a marathon – not everyone wants to, and that's okay – but perhaps you've seen people powering by on your way to work and felt you wanted to do that too, or have the ability to. If you think you can't run because you're not the right body type, fitness or identity, then this book is for you.

For many years I've been fortunate enough to make a living out of being the voice in people's heads that helps to get them moving. I probably shouldn't be giving this away, but the secret is, my friend . . . it's actually *their* voice that keeps them moving, I'm just the narrator here to amplify it. So let's work on developing that voice of *yours . . . together*. It will help you feel fantastic, both inside and out.

I am a runner and a running coach. Some of you will know me as Coach Cory, helping you pick up the pace on your run or encouraging you to vibercise. I run and I coach people to run because I love running. It keeps me fit and healthy and helps my body move the way I want it to. But, more than that, what it's really done is helped me on the *inside*. Running has given me not only the ability to move with speed and strength but also the mental and spiritual health that has led me on a positive path in life, so I can truly say that running has given me everything I have.

I've been exercising for probably my entire life, but I've been doing it seriously since 2006, when I was incredibly fat – like really, really fat: with a big belly, a big gut. My friends nicknamed me Beefhead because I had a big head. People clearly thought the fat was making my head swell as I was living life in an unhealthy way, living on auto-pilot instead of connecting with life. Then one day, someone told me I would never run a marathon. I proved them wrong. Then 'Beef' became just 'Bit Beefy', and things began to change.

I want to tell you about that change, because I didn't just start running one day and have an easy, smooth journey. There were a few steps in between, and some revelations too, and I want to share them because I think they could help you. I think they could help anyone to improve their life with running, especially if you think running isn't meant for you.

I wanted to write this book and share it with you because when I look at the TV and the bookshelves, I don't see my reflection. I don't see me. I see tons of amazingly tall and slim white athletes, and the black men I see are shiny superheroes, not normal everyday black dudes who could live at the bottom of your road; I don't see anyone that I really, really relate to. I see lots of books written from another point of view but nothing that reflects the road I've travelled.

Not seeing myself made me doubt what I could do, what I was capable of, the places that I could belong. I pushed on through that, convinced myself that I was only constrained by what my body and mind believed it could do. To begin with, I ran because someone told me I couldn't. Then I carried on because running connected with something vulnerable deep inside me. It was scary, but freeing, and the more I ran, the more I was challenged not just physically but also mentally, and I wanted to keep feeling it. I am living proof that running is for everyone.

I wanted to write this book for the person I was, the old Cory, the lost Cory of 20-odd years ago, and I also wanted to write this book for the person I am today, the Cory who is the beneficiary of a love affair with running. While writing I have delved deep into painful places in the back of my mind I haven't visited in a while. I did it because I know there are people out there who need that honesty, painful as it might be, and sharing my experiences will show what running can do for you.

I wanted to write this book for the community that I represent, for the community that supports me and wants me to win because I am them and they are me. I wanted to write this book because there are so many young black men out there who don't know yet that it's okay to be vulnerable, that it's okay to cry; that it's okay to not be okay and to need something to hold on to. Running can help you learn that. I wanted to write this book because I know I would have benefited from reading this, benefited from understanding that how I was living wasn't good for me – all the bravado, all the 'I'm good' and 'nothing fazes me', followed by the emotional eating; stuffing my face with sweets, chocolate, cake and fizzy drinks, smoking and drinking, partying my life away, not sleeping enough and not look-ing in the mirror – and I mean really looking in the mirror.

I know now how much better it would have been if I'd understood that playing the tough guy, pushing down my feelings, and not mourning the death of my grandmother who raised me would end up harming me in more ways than I could comprehend. We all have our pain, and this was mine, but the way out can be the same. My gran passed away 20 years or so ago. I couldn't tell you what year or what month it was because in a very sad way, I have done all I can to erase her passing from my mind. I try and remember how she lived, how her living made me feel.

No one can carry or drag you, you have to start walking and then run towards what is good for you and what will help you flourish.

I've written this book because I want people to realise that fitness and running can be accessible. I want people to understand that it's fun, that it can be a release and a joy; that it's a gift. I want people to appreciate the benefits of community and how having good people with you on your journey can help. *But* I also want them to realise that ultimately a good path and attainable happiness is up to you. It's YOU who must make the decision to move forward. No one can carry or drag you; you have to start walking and then run towards what is good for you and what will help you flourish. And if that means finding a new community that has more of a positive impact on your life then it's a decision that you will have to make.

I've written this book because, although running has made me stronger, in doing so it has exposed old scars and left new ones. If I can help others find a tool like running to help manage their lives a little better, instil some order and purpose when they need it most, then I feel part of my job will be done.

I've written this book as many people still don't know that running can be for them, still don't think running is a cool, interesting thing to do, don't find running accessible or fully understand its benefits. I've written this book because I wanted to let people know it is for them. It is for us. The roads, the countryside, the paths, everywhere is open to us learning to love running. I wanted to write this book because I needed people to know that, if you let it, running can set you free in every single way.

In many ways, I don't think I'm necessarily the best person to write a book – I'm not a scholar or a great thinker of my age. But I know that I'm the best person to tell my own story. With a lot of help along the road, I have navigated my way from fat dude who ate masses of cake to runner, to one of the head running coaches and adviser to the biggest sports brand in the world and then on to one of the biggest companies in the world. I am the co-founder of London track club and running lifestyle brand TrackMafia, and for a time I hosted a podcast in a bathtub, called *The Tub Hub*, about mental health and help.

Running offered me structure and purpose, and that became the scaffolding and steadiness I needed.

None of this would have happened if running hadn't made me acknowledge my weaknesses, and this is what I'm passionate about sharing. It's about channelling negativity into positive change and showing how doing so makes life all the richer. Running offered me structure and purpose, and that became the scaffolding and steadiness I needed as I moved away from the chaos and rebuilt a life that worked for me.

I want people to know that with time, patience and commitment this is all achievable. I want people to know that anyone can do it; I want people to read my story and feel inspired. I want people to read my book and be motivated to move, to ask for help, to change their lifestyle for a healthier one. I want to help you start running and keep going. I will give you tips on running routes to explore as well as tips and tricks on how to make movement and running fun, because I know that one of the barriers to getting started is quite simply that people think it's boring. And I'll tell you what to do when you get up in the morning and your body and brain shout 'Oh no, not today!' (Because, I'll tell you a secret, I still have those days too.)

I want people to finish reading feeling roused to acknowledge that no matter how small the change it paves the way for huge and long-lasting differences. Every hard run makes the next run better and better.

I wanted to write this book because I believe that, although there is nothing special about me, my journey thus far has been a unique one. I wanted to write this book as I believe my story is relatable, one that many will understand and hopefully take encouragement from. Why? Because if I can do what I have done, anyone and everyone can. I will give you the tools to get up and running, share what I've learned – both the good decisions and the mistakes I've made so you can learn from my experience. I'll help you step it up when you're ready and instil in you a mindset that allows constant learning, bettering and knowing yourself and a desire to soak up new ideas like muscle memory. I believe we all have a duty to share our learnings with the next generation as well as the current one, and celebrate the power of running. So come and run with me; I look forward to seeing you on the road.

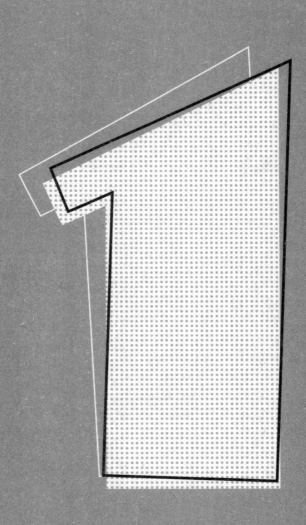

Run for Your Life

Why do people run, and why should you?

find it crazy nowadays to think that there was a time when I didn't run, a time when I lived my days without this movement. A time when I was blissfully unaware of the source of my unhappiness, and even unaware of my unhappiness at all. As you read this you may be thinking, what on earth does my unhappiness have to do with running? Let me explain.

You see, I often say that running is everything to me because running gave me everything. Running not only changed my life, but it also gave me the life I have . . . Let that sit for a little.

Is there anything in your world that has given you your life? Or changed you? Changed the way that you view the world, or changed the way that the world views you? I say this as life before I started running was very different. Let me take you back, *waaaaay* back, and set the scene for this unlikely story.

When I think about it, I floated through secondary school doing just enough to get by. Some subjects I had an interest in, but learning academically just seemed to bore me. I liked *doing* stuff, not sitting and listening. If there was a chance to get outside and do stuff, I was the first person to want to be involved. I also think that although at a young age I loved to learn, I liked to learn on my own terms, whether it be through doing or through discovery. I went to a government-funded secondary school in south-east London in the

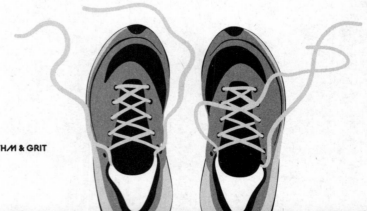

90s and at the time my school was home to an incredible jackpot of sports facilities: full-size grass sports pitches for football, hockey, rugby, athletics and cricket, twelve or so tennis courts, sports halls used for gymnastics, trampolining, netball, basketball . . . and there are probably a few sports that I have missed out.

I participated in every activity that was offered to me. I was sporty. Though I was terrible at basketball and swimming, I was okay at cricket, football, rugby and hockey. And I excelled at tennis and table tennis, and despite my fear of drowning I fell in love with water sports like Dragon Boating, canoeing and kayaking, as well as outdoorsy stuff like hiking and camping, and I proudly completed my Duke of Edinburgh award.

I only ever ran cross-country when I was asked to do so by teachers, as I always saw myself as more of a sprinter – there was just something special about being the fastest person on earth and I looked to GB sprinters Linford Christie and John Regis for inspiration. I wanted to be FAST like them. But I noticed that all the big-distance runners didn't really look like me, either in build or in complexion. They were long and lean and I was not.

If I'm honest the thought of running for such long periods of time never really appealed to me. Whenever I saw people running long distances they always looked so broken and wounded. From where I was sitting it seemed to be about enduring and suffering. Something that at that young age just didn't appeal (and still doesn't).

The point I'm trying to make is that sport and movement was encouraged and wasn't foreign to me. It was part of my day-to-day as a teen, a brilliant part of the schooling system – go to school, learn some things, play some sport.

I left school with an A in Drama but not much else. I was devastated, so upset, but I didn't know if I felt like that because I cared or because I knew it wasn't what my family expected. At the time I

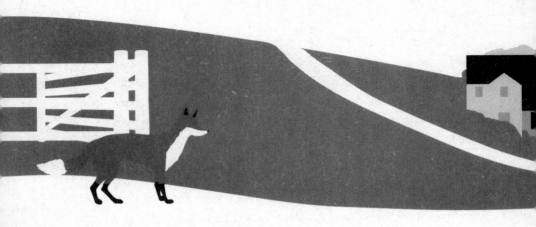

had no grand plan. No route pencilled out with goals. I remember showing my mum, Lyn, the results and her telling me that she was disappointed as she knew that I hadn't applied myself the way that she knew I could. But, she said, she wasn't worried about me; she knew I would find my way. She said, 'My son, whatever you choose to become, whatever you choose to do in this life, give it your all and be the best that you can be. You do that and you will be THE BEST at whatever you choose to be.'

These words stuck with me, words that I remember when I wake up every morning. Some might say that this was a cop-out, or that it wasn't a high bar that she set for me. I would argue that those words meant there was no bar or ceiling to hold me back. No pressure to stunt my growth or creativity. Just pressure to challenge myself to be better. Those words set me free and allowed me to explore, they allowed me to find myself, regardless of how long it took. Those words are why you are reading this now. So thank you, Lyn.

I enrolled in the college that was attached to my school and retook my maths and English exams, and instead of A levels I did an NVQ in Business Studies, walking away with a distinction.

But then, after all that activity and movement through school, I stopped playing sport, apart from the occasional five-a-side football match. It's something that seems to happen to a lot of people at that point in life. We leave a place where we are active every day

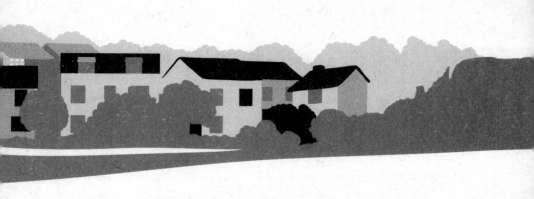

and fall into a world of inactivity, due to either a lack of facilities, a lack of finances to access those facilities or simply a lack of people to go to those facilities with.

I became a full-time journeyman going from job to job trying to find my way. Staying active didn't feel like a priority in 'real life', or so I thought at the time.

I worked as a demolition man, knocking through walls with sledge-hammers. I painted and decorated, plasterboarded, worked as a temp in accounts for the local authority, as a pizza delivery boy, a door-to-door salesman, a security guard, a club promoter, MC and host. I worked in pubs and pulled pints, I worked on the shop floor in retail, I was an enrolment and admissions officer at colleges and a customer service manager. And then finally I stumbled upon Westminster Council and got a job as a City Guardian.

This role was all about community, about going into neighbour-hoods in the borough of Westminster and helping residents with their problems. I was in Queen's Park, north-west London, and I worked with youth centres, churches, schools, rough sleepers, substance misusers, shops, charities, garden centres, radio stations and every-thing in between. Through this role I met a group of young people who wanted to start a football team but didn't have the means.

As I knew the area, I went into Moberly Sports Centre and asked to speak to someone about setting up a team. I was pointed to the sports development officer, a guy called Eugene Minogue, who told me I couldn't just set one up and coach kids because of health and safety and a need for qualifications. But . . . if I was really keen, and was willing to volunteer my services on one of his youth projects, he would pay for me to do my football coaching badges and everything else I needed to do to become a coach.

Of course I said yes, but at first I was confused. In my head, I was like, hold on, what? This dude is just going to pay for me to do this course? Just like that? And he's offering me this without even so much as a smile, he's not even being polite lol . . . No friendliness, no layering of lies, just very matter-of-fact, it was as if I had interrupted him and he'd come out to tell me to stop wasting his time. But that was Eugene, which is one of the many things I grew to admire about him. He didn't have time for airs and graces, but he had time to get stuff done or tell you that you weren't doing what you said you would get done.

Share your knowledge and spread the message.

So I carried on with my full-time job and agreed to work nights and weekends for the Sports Development Team at Westminster's Sports Unit. Eugene Minogue is now one of my best friends and I recognise now that this was my in, the little window to the future that I never knew existed. Eugene is a few years younger than me and was born and bred in Queen's Park, so he was very invested in doing his best to make the area a better place for his friends, family and community. We became such good friends that when he had his first child he was foolish enough to make me her godfather. (Hi Molly!)

I finished my football qualifications, started helping to coach a few local teams, then started playing in football tournaments with other coaches, locally and nationally. Then I completed a course which still to this day is the most important one I ever did.

It was called the CSLA, The Community Sports Leadership Award, and my tutor was Patricia Fairclough. What a legend — Patricia has been involved in basketball for well over 50 years and has an OBE awarded for services to the sport. She has spent her life nurturing thousands of the players, officials and volunteers that go on to help make not just basketball but all sports grow and flourish. She will always hold a special place in my heart as she is an older black lady who reminds me of my mum and gran. She spoke to me in a way that I would understand, and put me in my place several times. Though I was never rude, I always had questions.

The course was designed to help you develop the confidence to lead and run sessions for both young people and adults. It was about teaching you how to be a team player, and Patricia emphasised the importance of giving others an opportunity to excel, that things aren't always about *you*. She instilled in me the idea that knowing all the answers is great, but others knowing them too is even better. She inspired me to be better and think about more than just myself. SHARE YOUR KNOWLEDGE and SPREAD THE MESSAGE.

On the final day the exam was simple: entertain a sports hall filled with children with nothing but your wits and one or two pieces of equipment. On that day I learnt that kids don't care who you are or where you've come from, they care about *energy* and how much of it you have to share with them. They don't care about a perfect delivery or a well-articulated punchline, they care about *fun* – and lots of it.

I didn't realise what a big impact that course had on me until I started coaching for real in local youth centres and sports halls. I started to remember what it was like to play sport and move around. I had put on a *lot* of weight since school but I still had the muscle memory. So once I got going all I was really interested in was making sure that anyone who came to a session that I was at would have *fun*, fun and more fun. I began to lose a bit of weight – not a lot, because most of the job was about encouraging the kids to move themselves – but it was a start.

One of the projects that I worked on not only engaged with a hard-to-reach group of young people but also lowered the crime rate in the area that we working in. We made such an impression I was invited to speak at Buckingham Palace about the impact that sport had had on my life and the lives of the young people we were working with. It was a special moment for me, a signal that I was involved in something worthwhile that was making a difference.

A year or so passed during which I clocked up hours and hours of volunteering, and when a job came up working in Westminster's Sports Unit Sports Development Team as a Positive Futures co-ordinator I went for it. I switched teams and worked full time in a hybrid role that brought together elements of youth work, mentoring and coaching in a bid to use sports as tool to create better opportunities for young people to progress both in and outside of sports.

I loved my job and honestly woke up every morning thinking to myself, someone is paying me to do this, someone is paying me to play sport and work with young people. I thought life couldn't get any better.

That was, UNTIL I FOUND RUNNING.

n the beginning it was just this thing that I stumbled upon. Yet now it's at the heart of everything I do. In April 2006 I was 27 years old and I had been working at Westminster for a few years. I was stood watching the London Marathon for the first time. I remember thinking how strange it was that I had lived in London my entire life, but it had taken me nearly 30 years to physically go and see the race myself. A race that I had seen so many times on television. I guess it was the first time that I had a real reason to go in person.

I was with my mentor, boss and by now good friend Eugene, along with some other friends from the office who had all come out to cheer. We were waiting for our friend and work colleague Sam Bell to come charging through with a smile on her face so we could give her sweets and drinks, and of course scream and chant her name. It's what you do when people are running. You can't power their legs for them so you give them what you can.

She came flying along and looked like she had only been running for a few minutes, when in actual fact she'd been going for hours.

I found the whole experience so uplifting, feeling all that positive energy emanating from the streets, from the people, from the city. Some people weren't even there to cheer for anyone they knew, they just felt like they should be out there cheering anyone and everyone that ran by. There's something about cheering for strangers – it's like you're giving them a piece of you to help them on their journey.

Being at the marathon reminded me a little bit of a festival. It wasn't quite a carnival, but there was definitely a buzzing festival vibe. It was there, full of all that positive energy, that I declared to my friends that I would run the marathon the following year.

The laugh my friends let out when I said that I was going to take up running is probably exactly what made me do it. Because if I hadn't been serious when I opened my mouth, I became deadly serious when I opened

I found the whole experience so uplifting, feeling all that positive energy emanating from the streets.

my ears and heard a lot of:

'Bruv, are you sure?'

'Bruv, you eat a *lot.*'

'Bruv, I bet you won't.'

So, to all of you who 'bruvved' me, thank you for your inspiration. And for the few of you who said 'Cor, you got this', THANK YOU TOO.

So, at first, I ran because someone told me I couldn't. I wanted to prove that I could – to myself, to others, to the world. I wanted to be like those people running the marathon with big smiles on their faces, surrounded by screaming, shouting and cheers. I wanted to be able to move effortlessly and be happy about doing it.

I must admit it definitely got harder before it got easier, but I stuck with it, and I'm going to tell you how I started and all the things I did right (and all the things I could have done better) in the next chapter. For now I'll just say I made progress, but not as much as I thought I would, or as much as I wanted to. The question is, was this because I wasn't trying hard enough? Or because I had set myself unrealistic goals? And what kept me going?

After consulting the World Wide Web and some friends who knew more about running than I did, I came to understand that prior to running a full marathon one should run a half marathon to get some race experience and of course to cover the distance. So after I started running I signed up for what had been dubbed the biggest half marathon in the UK and second biggest in the world – the Great North Run, which was held in Newcastle.

arrived in Newcastle for my first half marathon *completely* unprepared. I mean, don't get me wrong, I had been running and training, but I had also been doing a lot of eating to fuel my training, and hadn't been covering the distances in train-ing that I needed to be ready. I say this as, looking back, I now know

I really didn't need a giant bowl of pasta to run two miles, but hey, I thought I was CARBO LOADING. A common mistake, I might add. I also now know that if I struggled to run a 10k without being at death's door I should have realised that doubling the distance might cause some problems, but no one could fault my commitment to getting to the start line.

Eugene and Sam joined me. Sam was the person who had originally inspired me to run, so it was only fitting that she be there to see me try.

This race was crazy for a number of reasons. It was crazy because I'd never done it before. Now it seems like the norm, but back then running in a race with another 35,000 people seemed crazy. Running along a closed motorway or dual carriageway seemed crazy. But it was crazy mostly because it was the first time I realised that running was doing something to not just my body but my mind as well.

I had been on runs before when my mind started to wander but I had always fought it, I had always done my utmost to shift my attention to things that I actually wanted to think about, things that I actively wanted to process, things that would help me deal with whatever my body was physically going through.

But this was different, this wouldn't shift. I kept thinking about someone whenever I tried to slip into the ZONE. Now, how does one describe the Zone? In big words terms it's where your thinking is inversely proportionate to the stimulus of the environment, or in small words terms you slip into a state where all you can think about is what you need to do here and now, everything else is blocked out. It's where your Jordans, Lebrons or Williams go when they make their big shots.

Instead of finding the Zone I would find the

woman who raised me; I was thinking about my gran. I kept seeing her face, hearing her voice, either willing me on or just being there – present. It was like a live feed of memories was being beamed directly to my glasses and there was no off button. I lost count of the amount of times I stopped myself from crying. It wasn't until I was about a mile or so out from the finish line, just as you start to go downhill before you turn left onto the seafront, that I couldn't hold it anymore and I cried all the way till I crossed the line. I realised it was half happiness and half sadness. I kept thinking, I miss her so much, but she'd be so happy with me. I had finished my first race, my first half marathon, I had a medal and a smile and I was happy. And let me tell you now, I couldn't walk properly for days. But was it worth it? HELL, YEAH . . . This is when things really started to change.

During the Great North Run, I realised that I still hadn't mourned my gran's passing, but I had found something that *might* just help me do so. The thing about running is all you have is time. Think about it: when you are doing other things, you kinda have to be in that moment thinking about them, focusing on them. But when you run, especially if you are running for a long time, it can feel like having a TV in your mind and someone else has the remote, and they are controlling the channels. Unless you spend all your time and energy finding the remote control and learning how to control it, you spend all your energy switching the channel back to something that you want to watch. Many years have passed since that first run, and nowadays when I run I have that remote control firmly in my hand.

I couldn't walk properly for days. But was it worth it? HELL, YEAH.

For so long I had run away from this pain, this feeling that any minute I might think about her. But now I sought it out, now I wanted it to come, I wanted to deal with it. My gran raised me when my mum was back home in Guyana, South America, working. She looked after me and my sister when my mum was back in London and at work. She picked me up from school, took me to church, cooked for me, bathed me and looked after me when I was sick. She was my rock.

When she passed 20 or so years ago I was in my twenties. It really did a number on me, as prior to her passing I hadn't really had to deal with a big loss like that. No one really wanted to talk to me about it and I didn't really want to talk to them about it, so it kinda just sat there. Fermenting. Slowly bubbling under the surface. After her passing I realised I'd have random bouts of real anger, then real sadness. Then the two combined. That just made me push people away and turn myself into this person that was void of any emotion, unless it was anger. As my little sister tells me, don't forget anger is an emotion, it's just not the one we like to talk about.

I was angry because I felt like she had left me without me saying goodbye. She was sick, and as the months passed and her condition deteriorated, I didn't want to say goodbye to someone who didn't look or feel like the strong person who looked after me when *I* was sick. I couldn't bear to see her like that. Then at the funeral when I saw her in that open casket it was so *final*. What upset me the most was that it wasn't how I wanted to remember her, and I know that it's not how she would want to be remembered. She was a fierce black woman who loved me. And that love I carry everywhere with me. If she could see what I'm doing now, she'd smile – she always said I had potential. ☻

remember listening to people talk about the *runner's high*, what it was like to get there, to feel it. They spoke about it like it was some kind of nirvana. If I'm honest, I wasn't convinced. At least I wasn't until it came. I had had the waves of sadness but never one of complete happiness or joy. But now, now, now it came. Running connected my physical self with my internal self. I felt complete, and now I could have this feeling whenever I ran.

It was some time after I was back in London running through Green Park when I felt it again. I was doing a 10k around the Royal Parks. It was a loop that I was familiar with, one that I had always enjoyed. Though you were in the city, you were still surrounded by trees and greenery. It was autumn, the fallen leaves were everywhere, and I knew rain was coming. As time had passed I'd grown to love the rain because for whatever reason it made me feel like a badass. It felt like I had chosen to be out when the elements were against me. I heard the sky open up in the distance and just waited for it to arrive . . . and boy oh boy did it arrive, it was like a scene out of a movie. It was as if someone had screamed *'Action!'* and they had turned on the tap in the sky, just the right amount of rain for it to be emotive. Just enough headwind for me to feel it. I felt like I was in *Hero* when Jet Li is preparing to duel. It's like everything is in slow-mo but you are still moving at speed. You get this weird tunnel vision, it feels like you are floating and in some way your body and everything else around it is connected. Your heart is pumping subtly in the background, your breathing is loud but merging with the sound of your footsteps and the ground beneath them. All of this combined with the battering of the rain makes for the perfect storm. And that's exactly what it created.

That beautiful moment in time was

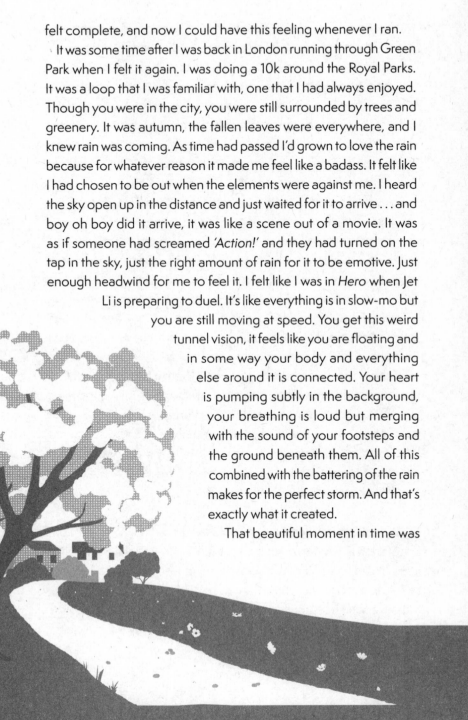

when I truly realised I had more. At that very moment I felt unstoppable, like I could go on forever. And it's this message that I want to share.

Each individual has their own journey to follow and yours will undoubtedly be different to mine, but as with most things in life you will find many similarities – we all breathe, we all move and we all need love, acceptance and understanding.

Whatever your reason for running, as long as you are getting what you need from it, it's doing its job.

At times it's hard to understand what is meant by 'doing its job'. For me it means giving you whatever you need at a particular moment and time. Some say that every run has a purpose, and I wholeheartedly agree. There will be days when you need a run to blast out all the nervous energy you have, days you need a run to help you smile, days you need to run just because that's what you need to do, that's what it says on your plan. There will be days when you just have an urge to run, and days when others will ask you to come. There is no right reason, only the run.

I found that these runs began to help me with my life outside of running. After my runs I felt invigorated, I felt alive, like someone had plugged me into the mains, I was just *buzzzzzing* and filled with energy. Many of the barriers that I had spent years mass producing and strategically placing around me were slowly but surely coming down. I found that I was far more open with people, far more forthcoming with information about my life. It might sound silly, but

It feels like you are floating and in some way your body and everything else around it is connected.

running actually helped me be a nicer person. I was more in tune with my emotions, more willing to listen, more willing to speak, but most surprising of all I was willing to both *give* and *take* HUGS. I was never a big hugger, it always felt too close, too personal, too invasive. I found that being more in tune with myself meant I was able to be more in tune with the world. That confidence and openness made me more approachable, some might even say more likeable. The little guy that had been hiding for so long started to pop his head out from behind the fence, and to my surprise he was welcomed with open arms, both by me and by the rest of the world.

The strange thing about life now is that it wasn't always like this. I didn't always know what was going on my head, I had no idea to be honest, I knew it was working but I hadn't quite got to the bottom of all the 'code' that was running in the background.

That was until I let go.

Since letting go, since that breakthrough moment on the Great North Run, and the clarity of that day in the rain in Green Park, running has become my guru. It's now where I go to think and where I go to see things clearly. Running gives me the confidence to do many things and, without it, I wouldn't have experienced all that I have. Without running I would be someone else.

So when people ask me what motivates me to run, the answer is: LIFE. Life is what motivates me to run, life is what motivates me to move. I want to live and I want to explore.

I want to continue growing, and that spark came from running.

You see running didn't just give me cardio, it gave me *cardio confidence* – it helped me to love, appreciate and accept myself so much more. I never really thought that self-acceptance was something that I needed to work on, but the more I ran the more time I had to think. The more I battled out on the road and broke down and failed, the more I said *THIS WILL NOT BEAT ME* – the more resilient I became. Some might think that that resilience is only used when you are running, but you'll find that that goodness finds its way into the rest of your life.

I saw noticeable changes in how I looked and how I felt. It was easier to move around and I started to wear clothes that I hadn't felt comfortable in before. This new-found positivity had all come from my improving health and my new relationship with my body. It gave me autonomy, real confidence about decisions I was making in my life. It improved my mental health, because those days when I used to feel like I couldn't be bothered with the world began to come far less frequently. I began to grow as a person because I had a goal, I had a challenge, something to motivate me. I'm not saying I didn't have a reason to get out of bed before, of course I did. But now it seemed bigger, more important. It created a domino effect. Through personal growth came more positive relationships, both with old friends and new – new friends I made through my new hobby, who were also on a journey. With their help I gained environmental mastery, that feeling where you think or even know that your body can do anything you ask it because you've done it before.

Running late for a train? No problem, I'll jog, or if I feel like it, I'll run and won't feel like everyone's looking at me when I battle my way through the closing doors. I won't be embarrassed as I won't be breathing heavily and sweating profusely.

These are the things that used to go through my head. Running helped me to be happy with myself and happy living in my own skin, so now when people ask I tell them. I run because I don't want to go back to being that dude who was lacking direction and real purpose. That dude didn't know what was going on in his head because he was too scared to go in there and explore. He was too scared to

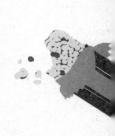

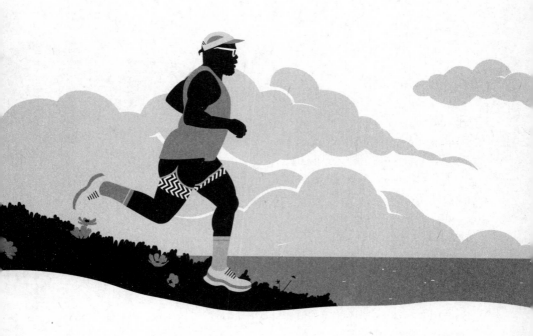

focus on making real change as failure scared him. Now my attitude is if you're not failing somehow, somewhere, there's room to try harder, room for growth. Running taught me to believe in myself, and in others. It taught me that I need to take care of myself, to eat well, to hydrate, to smile, to hug, to love, to feel emotion. It taught me it was okay to not be okay and that it was okay to share this with other people. Running is my safety net . . . Running saved me.

I'm not for one minute suggesting that what I do while running is for everyone. Many people I speak to run purely for performance, not for clarity or for feelings. Just know that regardless of why it is that you run, your reasons are valid.

There are days that I find myself heading out for a run with no distance or destination in mind, and I just let mind and body guide me. I let my mind wander, I sift through problems, through feelings, I think about projects that I'm working on. And sometimes magical ideas will appear, or I'll find answers for questions that I never knew I needed to ask.

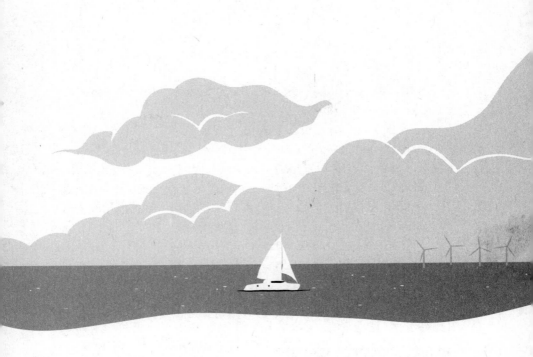

Over the years I have worked on fine-tuning these methods with a few simple exercises. Exercises that have helped me make little maps in my mind. In the beginning I would struggle to clear my mind as I tried to force thoughts out of my head, now I let them pass and not linger. It's like a map in my head or a web of connections, each interlinked but all focused on two things: peace and progression. Why not give it a try?

Either in your head or writing it down in a notebook, just ask yourself: right now, today, what things would help to bring you peace? And progression? Then when you've jotted them down make a mental note of those things and take them with you on your run and think about them. You'll find that maybe the answers you were looking for or hiding from might appear.

As I'm sure you are aware, there are also many people who run to compete for medals, silverware, times or records, or simply to run as fast as they can. I'm not saying that those who run for peace aren't interested in the science of running or how fast they are going, of course there is some crossover. The difference is the order in which our list is formed.

Some run for records and for medals, others run for weight management or as a means to stay fit for another sport. Whatever your reason, whatever motivates you, neither I nor anyone else has grounds to question it. We should simply congratulate you for persevering. Just like life, the simple act of putting one foot in front of the other is far from simple, it's an act of defiance.

It's an interesting one. When I look in the mirror and I'm unhappy about my body, I run to change it. Still, to this day there are times when I catch my reflection and I know there's work to be done. Regardless of how much work I do, the little sugar demon in me still calls, the lazy guy still says, *bruvvvvvaaa*, come sit on the couch and think about tomorrow. And when I listen to that call, I see a change in how I look and how I feel. But that will always be there, it's about putting things in place to combat those messages.

Everything that I need to overcome any obstacle is inside me if I can dig deep enough.

When I look in the mirror and I am overjoyed by my body, I run to maintain it. When I'm sad I run to clear my mind, yet when I'm happy I run to celebrate my happiness. Running has become this non-negotiable part of my life that I go to regardless of how I'm feeling. When I look at the full spectrum of emotions I don't think there's anything else that I do or have done that is there for me the way running is.

There are also times when I have no idea why I'm running. I just have an urge, a called nagging, niggling voice in the back of my head that says *run, go, run, go, now*, escape from this place. I used to think it was because I was scared of something, but I couldn't figure out what it was. At times that feeling comes from nowhere, like a wave. But like most waves, it passes. But then another will come.

It took a while for me to work this out but during this time I would say quietly to myself, FEAR NOT THE WAVE FOR THE WAVE IS WITHIN YOU. I used to say it to my long-time friend Flowers (his real name is Tom and I've known him ever since he turned up at my RDCWest road run one Monday night and proceeded to run a sub 5-minute mile barefoot on concrete around the park where we regularly did intervals) and to be honest, he was the only person at the time who got what I was talking about. Everyone else thought I was being ridiculous or purposely weird. But I'm okay with that, and to this day I find that phrase so empowering. I guess it's my way of saying I have nothing to fear but fear itself. Everything that I need to overcome any obstacle is inside me if I can dig deep enough. The question is always, how deep am I willing to dig?

This is how I find BALANCE, this is how I maintain balance in my life. This is why I run, and one of the many reasons why – if you are willing – YOU SHOULD RUN TOO.

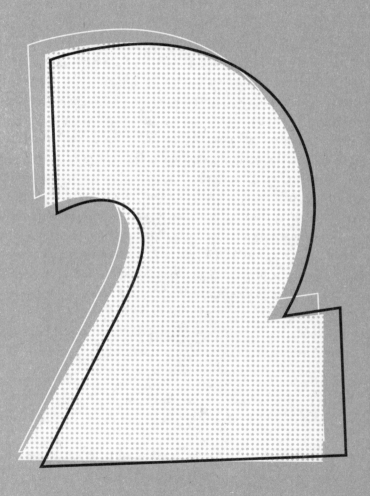

Start at the Beginning

To the end of the road and back

You might think to yourself, ahhhhhh, it's easy for him to say 'you should too', Coach Cory is now at a place where things are no longer hard. I really do wish it was that simple, I really do wish every run that I went on was one that I was excited about, 100 per cent committed to and once I was out there, a run that I floated along at a pace that felt easy and free.

But the truth is, my friends, *that's not the case*. I would say that the only difference between me and you on these runs is I have a little more experience and knowledge, and maybe the understanding that at some point on my run, things *might* start to feel a little better, or they might *not*.

The purpose of me saying this is not to scare you or to make you put this book down or give up. I am telling you this because I want you to be realistic and understand that this is a journey with no destination or real end point. It's a journey with stops on the way that will give you some of the tools to help you better manage the next part of your journey, or to help you be better equipped to revisit a destination or stop on your journey that you have visited before.

You see, in the beginning what I really needed was a book like this that told me it was okay to get better gradually and that every minute spent moving was a win. It's okay for the first run to feel really, really hard. That is normal. Your first ever run won't feel easy because you've never done it before! I needed a book that told me it wasn't just about having the gear, but that it was better to have an idea of what I wanted to achieve. And just to be clear, when I say achieve, I'm not talking about grandiose expectations. The achievement could be as simple as I WANT TO RUN. It doesn't matter how far, how long for, how often or how fast. The simple act of running, of putting one foot in front of the other, is enough. No need for anymore. If that's your wish and that's where you are starting from, don't be afraid to own that.

It took me a while to work it out but I am glad I did; I am glad I stuck with it as it means I can share it with you. When you start, try and think about *your* starting point – this is the best measure of achievement. Forget about other people, other places – FORGET! Think about ending each session a little bit better than you started, and remember better doesn't always mean faster. If you keep that in mind, the rest will follow.

The morning after running the Great North Run for the first time I genuinely felt like I had been hit by a train. I had my *aha* moment and something opened up in my brain during that run and it was amazing, but it didn't remove the physical effects of what I had put my body through. I had run 13.1 miles or 21k and my muscles were so sore I was walking backwards down a flight of stairs, moaning and whinging about how much pain I was in. How my body was cramping, how I couldn't stand straight. I kept saying: how long will this last? I said, listen, isn't DOMS (Delayed Onset of Muscle Soreness) supposed to be worse on day two? If this is day one, I may need care tomorrow as I'm not sure I can deal with more.

I thought to myself, *how on earth* am I going to run double the distance if I am in this much pain now? At that point I had to give myself a little pep talk as I realised that when I started there was no way I would have been able to cover half the distance I had just run.

For some strange reason I was already telling myself I couldn't do something in the future, even though I had already proved to myself I could do more than I thought I could. My question was why? Why even before trying did I question the possibility? I sidestepped that negative thought and replaced it with a positive one. I now said that if I kept with it, if I worked hard – or should I say if I worked a li'l harder and really committed – I would eventually get there.

I think back to the beginning, and I ask myself what would have made things easier for me? What would make things easier for *you*?

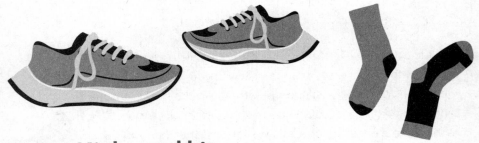

Kicks and kit

Step one is to get yourself **a comfortable pair of trainers**. Nothing more challenging than that. Get yourself a pair of trainers that you like the look of. They don't have to be catwalk ready, but you should like them. I suggest getting a pair of proper running trainers as they will offer you the support and comfort that you need. Yes, it's true that people all over the world run barefoot or in minimalistic shoes that weren't built with running in mind, *but* if you would like to start your running journey in comfort and they are accessible to you, I'd suggest getting running shoes.

As I am sure you are aware, comfort is very subjective, so find something that feels right for you instead of relying solely on other people's opinion. Of course, ask around, use the World Wide Web to dig into what's available and at what cost, but ultimately the decision is yours. I'm not going to tell you what brand or style is best, just that it should FEEL GOOD TO YOU.

We all prioritise comfort features differently, so I suggest going to a specialist running shop and trying on a bunch of shoes from different brands. Or, if you already have a particular brand in mind, go to the store owned or operated by that brand – whether that be a Nike Town, Adidas, Asics, Brooks, Saucony, New Balance, Hoka or ON running. If not endless, the options are plenty.

Ask the specialist that's attending to you to give you a wide variety of shoes to try on. Tell them how much you would like to spend and ask them why they recommend trying on this shoe in particular, then ask yourself the following questions. (If you need to, make notes,

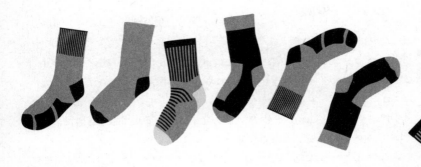

and don't be afraid to take your time. This is not only a financial investment but an investment in your future comfort.)

» How does the shoe fit?
» How much cushioning does it have?
» How much support does it offer?
» How stiff is it?
» How breathable is it?
» How long will it last?

And of course the questions some tend to forget:

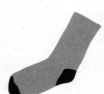

» DO I LIKE THE LOOK OF THESE SHOES? WILL I BE HAPPY TO WEAR THEM?

Because if I think they are ugly and make my feet look like hooves (laughs loudly), am I actually going to be happy wearing them? Or will this become a reason for me to not put them on?

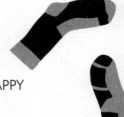

I am speaking from experience here. I have used that excuse many times, but now that I am older and wiser, I know better. Find the balance between function and fashion and it's even more reason to get out there and smile. If you aren't too concerned with being at the forefront of technology and fashion, I suggest asking for sale items of products that are either being discontinued due to a new model coming out, or for last year's model. Just know that if you choose that route when it comes time to get a *new* pair of your beloved shoes, they may have stopped selling it, or you may have to go hunting for it on the Web or in outlets.

Once you are done with the kicks, if you would like to invest a little more, ask them for a pair of **running socks**.

Why running socks? Well, they are built a little differently to the socks we wear to work, to weddings or the cluuuuuub. They are designed to help reduce blisters and wick away the moisture and sweat that builds up while you're running, and they offer a little extra layer of comfort to your feet.

I am not for one minute suggesting that you cannot or will not get blisters with running socks, but you are far less likely to. When I first started running I ran in socks that were not made for running and I paid the price. They rubbed everywhere, so I had blisters on my heels, the soles of my feet, in between my toes – *everywhere* – which either meant I couldn't run until they healed or my run was uncomfortable and a lot harder than it needed to be. All because, at the time, I thought running socks were a complete waste of money.

Now you're chomping at the bit and you are ready to hit the road, what should you wear? I hear you cry. Once again, SOMETHING COMFORTABLE.

If you are already active you will no doubt have some kit you can put on to run in, like shorts or tights for the lower half and for your top half a T-shirt or long sleeve, or if it's a little chilly a jacket and a hat.

If you are starting from scratch you can do what I and many others did, which is dig around your wardrobe and drawers and find something to run in, whether it's old shorts or tracksuit bottoms, and a battered old T-shirt – anything you are comfortable running in. An old band T-shirt or something you cook in, an old hoody you normally snuggle up on the couch in. *In the beginning it really doesn't matter.* You don't need the latest, snazziest, brightest bit of kit for your first run, in a few weeks or months that stuff will be there waiting for you. If it's cold make sure to wrap up warm, if it's wet be sure to wear a waterproof. I'll say it again, this is your first run, you do not need all the specialist kit unless the weather demands it. (More to come on kit later.)

Once you've got the kicks that you need, I suggest unboxing them, putting them on and getting used to how they feel on your feet. Something I found very helpful was just sitting in my kicks and kit and thinking about where I would like to run and imagining the feeling of joy when getting there.

Why not take a minute and try that now, even if you're not in your kicks. Close your eyes – or keep them open – and imagine yourself running, smiling, enjoying yourself, embracing that feeling of accomplishment. What are your surroundings like? What can you smell? What does it feel like to win? And when I say win I simply mean stepping out of your front door to go for your first run. *But,* just to be clear, *not* going for a run is not the equivalent of losing, you are simply still on your way to winning. It's a MINDSET.

This is your first run, you do not need all the specialist kit unless the weather demands it.

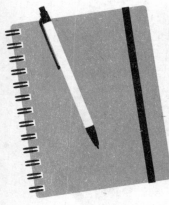

Pick a time

Now that you have thought about the feeling, it might be time to commit to it. Pick a day and a time that you want to run and put it in your diary or calendar if you need to, but remember there's no pressure.

When starting out it's much easier to incorporate new movement into your day-to-day activities – your walk for coffee or walk to the shops could now start with a little run. You could run to lunch or to the gym, or get off the train or bus one stop earlier or later.

Also, when deciding what time you want to run, think about the kind of person you are. Are you a morning person who wants to get things done when it's quiet on the streets so you can enjoy the rest of your day? Are you a lunchtime runner, squeezing it in during your break? An early evening runner, either after work or before dinner? Are you a late night runner who wants to look forward to it for the whole day? Or do you have all the time in the world and can run whenever you like?

I am asking all of these questions as it took me quite a while to work out that if I am given the opportunity to choose, I never choose to run first thing in the morning. I'm just not a morning person; I need a little while to wake up and prefer to run between the early evening and late at night. *But* it's something that I have had to get used to. Most organised races, especially the ones over longer distances, tend to be held first thing in the morning. Just something to think about when you're planning.

It's great to start new things like these at the beginning of the week or month, but just as great to start whenever you are ready. If it's a Thursday night at 9.03 p.m. after watching the latest episode of your favourite show, then that's the time for you to go.

Set your intention

Your 'intention' can be time based or distanced based – run to the bottom of the road and back, make it around the block, or run for 30 seconds to 1 minute and walk for the same length of time 2 to 10 times. As you know, my first run was all about getting to the bottom of the road. I made it, and built up from there.

Once your intention has been set, SET TWO MORE. The first is what I and a few others like to call the GOLD intention. That's the one that's capitalised, the medal that you really, really want. The next two are the SILVER and BRONZE intentions. So if your Gold is to run to the end of the road, a Silver might be to run halfway down the road, and a Bronze might be to run to the first lamp post.

A little later, your Gold intention might be a whole mile, Silver might be three-quarters of a mile and Bronze might be half a mile. You get the idea.

It's good to set these other intentions. What you don't want to happen is you run further than you've run before or than you ran a few minutes ago, but because you didn't cover the time or distance that you planned to, you consider yourself a failure, or feel like you have let yourself down, when that just isn't the case. You still achieved something, something more than if you had stayed at home and said *not today*.

Just think of yourself as an Olympian lining up to race: the fact that you are at the Olympics at all is a big deal in itself, so getting a medal is an even bigger deal, even if it's not gold. It means you worked but there's still work to be done.

Prepare

You have counted down the days, it's the day before your first run. Make sure to hydrate, eat well, but not more or less than you would usually, and – most importantly! – get your 8-plus hours sleep. Believe it or not, in this running game **sleep** is your secret weapon, your underrated superpower.

Whether you are running first thing in the morning or when you get in from work, make sure to lay your **kit** out ready so you don't have to hunt around looking for it. The dream is to keep the stress level *lowwwww* before you head out. If you're planning on running from elsewhere, make sure your bag's packed and ready to go.

Visualise, visualise, visualise – POSITIVE thoughts. I cannot stress this enough. Some people say get out your own head. I say NO, get *in* your head and tell yourself you're awesome and you are going to get it done. When you're putting on that kit, you are a superhero suiting up getting ready to go out and make *your* world a better place, and in doing so making the *whole* world a better place. Because when you smile, guess what? The whole world smiles with you.

Now, just to be clear – in the same way that you have set your intention for this run, you also need to set your expectations. You need to acknowledge and understand that your first run could well be terrible, and you may well hate it. But that is not a reason to not try, or to stop trying.

I am saying this because MINE WAS. My first run was awful; my back hurt, my legs hurt, and it felt like I was carrying bags of shopping around my midriff. I caught my reflection in a car window and thought I looked like a bear that had had one too many beers on a night out. I was so embarrassed and I thought to myself: Nahhhh, hold on, how was it so hard for me to run to the bottom of the road and back, why am I breathing like this? Is this what it's supposed to feel like? Am I supposed to be struggling for air? Searching for a seat? A pit stop maybe? And sadly, the answer is yes. If like me you haven't taken care of your body, or you're unfit, or returning from injury, trying this running thing for the first time, testing your body and or pushing your *current* limits, then, yes, there will be some discomfort that you may well have to embrace and push through.

When you're putting on that kit, you are a superhero suiting up getting ready to go out and make your world a better place.

Without venturing or exploring outside your comfort zone, your potential for growth is greatly reduced.

Just to be clear, there is a big difference between **pain** and **discomfort**, and it's for you to work out where those lines begin, end, and of course, *blur*.

I treated running like I have treated many TV programmes that have been recommended to me over the years. If I made my decision after the first episode or two I probably wouldn't have stuck it out, but there were people who had been there before me who said, you will love this, just get past the first few and you'll see why we do what we do. So I did. And without that gift from those who had walked this road before, I would have missed out.

So, remember, it will get EASIER, it will get BETTER, and you will become STRONGER.

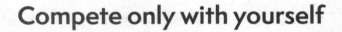

Compete only with yourself

Remember where you are starting from and don't compare yourself to anyone else. Not to the Olympians you see floating freely on the telly, not to your friends who have been running longer than you. And most certainly do not listen to the negative opinions of those who wish to bring you down because they are not willing or brave enough to join you.

This was something that I encountered a lot. A lot of opinions, judgement, advice and commentary from people who have never run before and are in the same place as you. For now, let's call them 'back seat drivers' or 'armchair coaches' and for now and forever more, unless they have something insightful, helpful, inspirational or positive to say: IGNORE them, or use their comments and lack of tact as fuel for not only your run but your journey.

Warm up

Now then, I would suggest doing a warm-up before kicking things off. You don't have to do it, but it helps to set habits and routines like this early in the game and it's great for getting the body and mind ready for exercise. It gets the blood pumping and activates the muscles you'll need to perform at your best. Do each of these exercises for 15–30 seconds, depending on your fitness level – you'll know what's right for you.

Try these warm-up drills:

1

LUNGES FORWARD AND BACK

Feet hip width apart, chest up. Take a big step forwards with your right foot. Lower until both your knees are bent at 90 degrees and your front thigh is parallel to the floor. Come back to a standing position. Repeat on the other side. Then go for a reverse lunge. Take a big step back with your right foot. Lower until both your knees are bent at 90 degrees and your back thigh is parallel to the floor. Return to a standing position. Repeat on the other side.

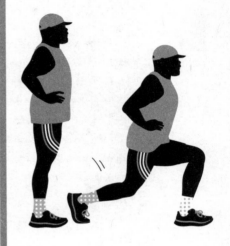

2

HEEL FLICKS AND LEG SWINGS

Think of trying to hit your bum with your heel, then loosely swing your leg up trying to reach the sky.

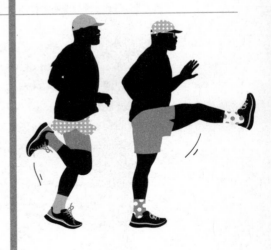

3

FAST FEET

Stand in a position as if you were trying to prevent a toddler from running past you, with your feet shoulder width apart. Come up onto the balls of your feet. Now move as if there are grapes beneath you and you are trying to squash them quickly to make wine or grape juice.

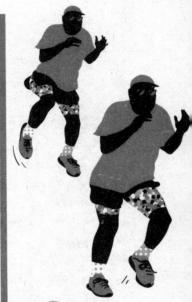

4

HIGH KNEE- OR A-KICKS

Stand straight, with your feet shoulder width apart. Think HEAD UP, KNEE UP, TOE UP when doing this. Bring one of your knees up to waist level with the other leg left standing. Slowly land on the balls of your feet and switch legs. Build in pace as time passes. With fast feet the goal is to crush the grapes over time. With high knees the goal is to crush them quickly.

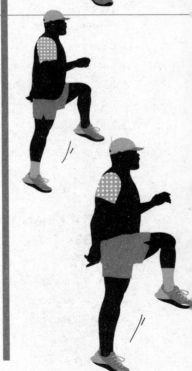

5

ARM WINDMILLS BACK AND FORTH AND ARM DRIVE

Think aggressive standing backstroke, followed by an unorthodox front crawl. Then think performative arm driving. Elbows at 90 degrees, pumping and driving backwards and flying forwards.

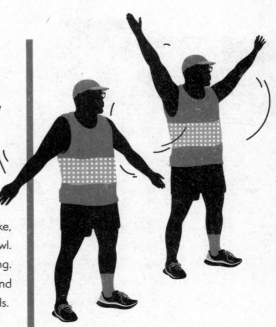

6

SQUATS AND OPEN DOOR/CLOSE DOOR (HIP OPENERS)

Think sitting on a chair then getting up; as you get up, you bring your leg up, flash your inner knee, then hide it away. Or open the door and close the door.

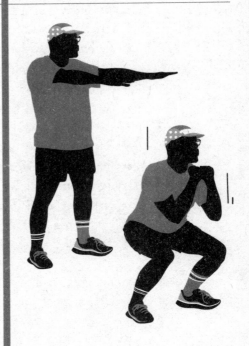

Now take to the door and if you can, close your eyes . . . Take a few deep breaths and listen to the sounds that surround the space. Roll your shoulders front and back and get rid of any tension that you might be carrying up there, then repeat after me:

➤➤ I GOT THIS – IT AIN'T GOT ME.
➤➤ FEAR NOT THE WAVE, FOR THE WAVE IS WITHIN ME.

Say it once, twice, three times, either in your head or OUT LOUD, gradually getting louder and louder as your fill your space with your GOOD ENERGY. The energy that makes you *really believe* that you've got this. Head out the door and carry as many of these thoughts with you as you wish. One of them, or all of them:

➤➤ Remember why you're there or for whom.
➤➤ Remember your intention.
➤➤ Remember this is your first time, *not* your last time.
➤➤ Remember that it could feel terrible, but that is *not* a reason to not do it again.
➤➤ Remember your goal.
➤➤ Remember how far or for how long you wanted to go.
➤➤ Remember your Bronze, Silver and Gold.
➤➤ Then just LET GO.
➤➤ Let the road take YOU and YOU it.
➤➤ Fly. Float. Be free.

Breathe and acknowledge that with these few steps you have chosen to be better, you have chosen to put yourself out there, to challenge yourself, to try something new – and most importantly you were willing to be vulnerable.

On the run

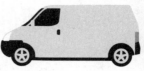

When you're moving, settle into a pace that feels natural, that feels right, a conversational pace. It doesn't matter how fast or how steady that pace is as long as it's yours. If a 105-year-old passes you, sipping tea, carrying shopping while pushing a buggy with twins in, IT DOES NOT MATTER. You are not to compare yourself to others, only to yourself.

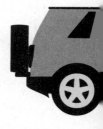

Find **markers** out there to help pass the time. In the beginning my markers were anything that I could find: get to the bottom of the road, to the next house, the next red or yellow car, run till I see another person walking their dog – *anything* I could find to make myself feel like I was making progress, winning at my own little game. A decade or so later, nothing has changed. I am still looking for markers to help motivate me to keep moving or give me reason to relax, and I find them wherever I go. And so can you.

Remember this is your run, your time to explore what feels right. There's a difference between pain and discomfort. So work out what it is. I have always viewed pain on a run as indicating that something has gone wrong or is going wrong, so I must stop and find out what. Discomfort is, I'm doing something right but it's hard and uncomfortable. But if I persevere, I can do it. The question is, for how long? Remember each run is a learning experience and an opportunity to find out a little more about yourself.

As you start to get a few more runs under your belt, ask yourself, did you feel a little less achy after? Before or during? Did you recover a little more quickly? Were you able to have a conversation, or sing? These are all signs that your cardio is improving. Did you get to your marker a little quicker than before? Did it feel easier? Was the smile a little brighter? Never forget, progress is measured in so many different ways.

The finish

Once you've finished, congratulate yourself, tell yourself how awesome you are, how amazing you are for getting out there and challenging yourself, doing something different and believing in your own ability.

Then ask yourself, how was that, how do I feel? Not how quick did I go. Give me something emotive. I'm not trying to steer you away from measuring your times. But I am trying to get you to not always attach emotion or feelings to numbers.

If you so wish, write down how your run made you feel. What was the weather like? What did you see on the run? Did you find the run challenging or easy? If you are not the writer type, try and remember these little patterns and learnings, as they are some of the things that will help you improve as a runner. They will help you to enjoy running a little more and help you get the best out of it.

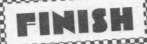

The next run, and the next

Whatever time or distance you covered, do the same every other day for 1–2 weeks until the distance or time that you picked feels noticeably easier than when you began. It feels like light work in comparison to when you began. It feels like you could sing while doing it.

Once you've done it a few times, see if your body feels like it could do a little more. You will know when it feels right for you. When it does, add a little more time or distance, maybe another 10 to 20 per cent. Whatever feels right. BUT NO MORE THAN THAT.

When I first started, I tried to run in two-week cycles as I always wanted a rest day in between runs. A cycle would look something like this:

» Monday – Wednesday – Friday – Sunday – Tuesday – Thursday – Saturday (back to Monday).

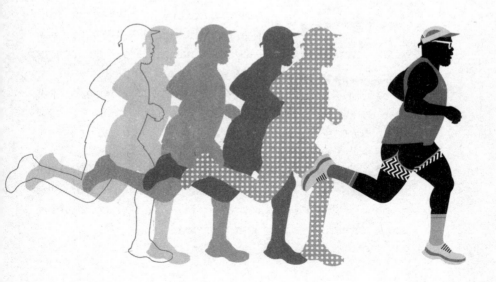

I know many people prefer to have the same schedule every week, so this works for a lot of people:

➤ Monday – Wednesday – Friday – Sunday (back to Monday).

To make it a little easier on the body, run early on Sunday and late on Monday as that will give your body a little more time to recover. To make it harder, run late on Sunday and early on Monday as that will give the body less time to recover.

In this new world of social media the question is always to share or not to share, and my response is it's entirely up to you. If you believe that sharing with your friends and strangers, or friends you haven't made yet, will give you a little boost, or you might be able to get some encouragement, help and advice or find a community – or, better yet, build your own – then tell people about your journey and your new-found love. *But* if you feel like there's a chance that someone might say something insensitive that might impact you negatively, then keep your joy to yourself and those close to you. It's sad that there are people out there who wish to be mean, but it would be irresponsible of me to not acknowledge that they exist.

I must say it was the very first run that felt the worst. Every run afterwards felt a little bit better.

In the beginning I had a rule: I would only share my journey with those whose numbers I had. That rule didn't last long, but in the beginning it helped me grow without the interference of others, especially while I trained for my first marathon.

Starting might be hard, but it also might not be. I must say it was the very first run that felt the worst. Every run afterwards felt a little bit better, even if sometimes harder as the challenge slowly transformed from starting to carrying on the running journey. It is every bit worth it, and I suggest you continue to put one foot in front of the other and run until it starts to feel a little easier. Don't rush it, keep going, and one day you'll wake up and feel ready to step it up . . . if only a little bit.

My first marathon

I had just come off the back of a disappointing run at the Great North Run. I say disappointing as that's how I felt initially. I didn't get close to the time I wanted and my body felt like I'd been struck multiple blows by Thor's magical hammer.

But then I sat back and really thought about it. Time was truly irrelevant as I had just run my first half marathon, further than I had ever run before. Only a few months before, even the thought of covering such a distance was mind boggling. So I shifted my mindset to one of what I *did* do, not what I *didn't*.

There were still six or seven months to prepare for my full marathon after the emotional rollercoaster of a race that was the Great North Run. The bizarre thing is I knew exactly what I had to do to get ready for my first marathon, but I just never really got going. I didn't train enough, I didn't sleep enough, I didn't do any strength work, no yoga, not enough work on my balance, mobility or range of motion. I didn't really do any tempo runs (see Chapter 5), certainly no speed, I ate too much and put on even more weight – which I later found out isn't uncommon when training for a marathon. To sum it up, unbeknown to myself I did everything in my power to sabotage this race for myself, as I later realised. Most of us can get through a half marathon when we haven't done enough, but getting through a marathon when you haven't done what you're supposed to do is a FOOLISH, PAINFUL, HUMBLING experience. But it's one that if I could redo it a thousand times I wouldn't change. That pain is what made me dig deeper than I have ever had to, than I ever needed to.

Many of my friends knew I wasn't ready. There was lots of 'Bruv, isn't this running thing supposed to make you lose weight?' and 'How come you're heavier now?' I remember showing some friends my running outfit and them asking why I had so many layers. Why were there so many clothes? My response was, who knows what might happen out there . . . If things don't go the way I want them to, I don't really want to be out there wearing next to nothing, being scantily clad feeling all cold and exposed. They asked what the longest training run was that I'd done. Me, knowing full well I hadn't actually run any further than I did at the Great North Run. I had covered 21k, only half of the distance that I needed to cover. But I knew that this had to be done.

I went to the London Marathon expo and picked up my bib. In the back of my head I was thinking, defer, defer, defer . . . postpone, postpone, postpone . . . but even further to the back of my head was this little voice that said, they expect you to defer, they want you to fail, they don't think you can do it. Go out there and prove them wrong. So I did just that.

I went home, ate a lot of food, got my energy drinks and gels ready (see pages 88–9 about energy gels), got my kit ready, pinned my numbers on my vest, worked out how I was going to get to the start. Asked friends and family where they would be to cheer for me then switched off the lights and tried to sleep.

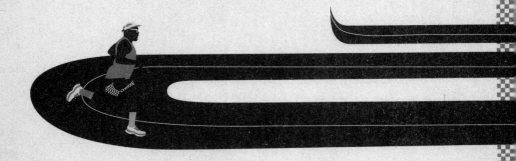

If I could use the eyes emoji, I would use it right here. There was no sleep, my eyes were wide open. Just thinking about the next day, race day, thinking about failure, thinking about my lack of readiness. And then it was morning. I honestly do believe I got two, maybe three hours' sleep, if that. This is not what I needed.

I made my way to the start line, said my goodbyes and see-you-laters to the fam, handed my bag in and waited. It was at that moment I felt so alone.

I realised that I just wasn't ready to do what I had set out to do, but also at that very moment I realised it was something that I had to do regardless. I didn't know that act would change me and the course of my life forever, I just went for it. I was so nervous, so panicked, and my head was filled with both positive and negative thoughts. It was like waves crashing through my mind. First it was: you're not ready for this, you can't do this, you're too slow, too overweight, haven't trained enough, why don't you just go back to bed and forget about it or do it another day.

It was like a duel between good and evil. Not too long after having those thoughts I got the fightback. Yes you can do this, you may

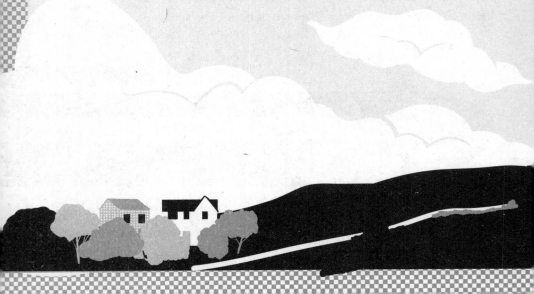

not have trained enough but you are going to finish by hook or by crook, to prove something to yourself, to prove something to your gran. And of course to prove something to all the naysayers who thought you were going to crumble into a ball and give up as you just didn't have the minerals for it. I realised that if I wanted this I had to FIGHT FOR IT – so fight I did.

Was the weight of the rest of the race weighing me down? Or was it the pies?

The first six miles were a joke, I thought, how does six miles feel like this? I just couldn't find a rhythm, it felt hard, harder than six miles had felt before. Or was the weight of the rest of the race weighing me down? Or was it the pies? If all I had to do was run six miles and have a nap it would be fine, as it felt like that was all I had in me. I've got 20 miles left, right?

I got to around seven miles and it started to rain. I got to eight miles and tried to jump over a puddle, as god forbid my feet get wet. I mistimed said jump, rolled my ankle and proceeded to scream in agony and panic about this race. At that time I had no idea what a

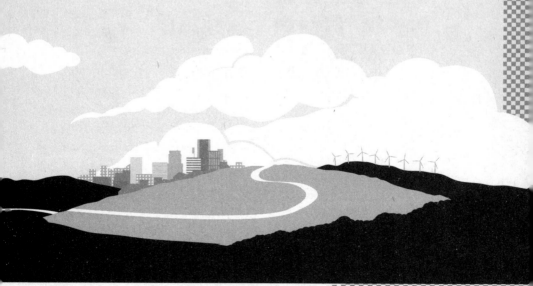

DNF (Did Not Finish) was. All I knew was even if I had to walk the remaining 18 miles I *would*.

After a while the pain eased off and I walked and ran the remainder of the race. The crowds were so supportive – people screaming my name, offering me sweets, drinks, gels, high fives, and it didn't matter what pace you were running. Their support and love was for everyone. When people saw me struggling they'd scream, 'You can do it man, keep going!' When people saw me cramping they helped me stretch. It's events like this that really restore your faith in humanity. Because, if you have no friends or family out there running or an interest in the sport, why would you give your day up to cheer on a random stranger?

Yes, there's noise, there are people cheering, music playing, but for that whole race I was alone in my head, alone in my thoughts. So everything that I had chosen not to think or talk about – and I mean *everything* – went through my head. It was like I had a free seven-hour counselling session, because that's how long it took me. Nearly seven hours.

> **It's events like this that really restore your faith in humanity.**

I realised that mentally I wasn't in the best place. There was a bunch of stuff that I hadn't addressed, that I pushed to the bottom of my being. Especially stuff around my gran's passing. I just hadn't mourned. And I didn't know how. I wasn't happy with most of the things in my life but I just kinda got on with it. What else do you do? Who do you talk to about stuff like that? Who do you trust? Who can you open up to that won't throw what you're saying in your face at some point? Who do you show that you're vulnerable? At that point, *no one*. It was just me and the road. Yes, I had had that *aha* moment when I ran the half marathon, but it wasn't the place that I had decided that I wanted to venture to willingly yet. But like clockwork, the deeper into the hole I got on my run the more I thought. The more I thought, the more I opened myself up to it. The more I struggled physically, the more my mind was flooded with thoughts about my gran. There were times when I honestly just wanted to pull the plug, and if I couldn't somehow cut the feed I wanted to grab the remote and change the channel. That's sadly not how it works. You have to do the work.

As I ran the final few hundred metres of the race, down Birdcage Walk, I saw my mum, Lyn, my li'l sis Janeen, my friends Katuchia, Ishmael, Clarkey, Eugene and the original inspiration for my very own 'Fight the Fat' campaign, my friend Sam. I waved, they cheered. I crossed the finish line and searched for somewhere to collapse and be with my thoughts. I was exhausted, both mentally and physically. Everywhere hurt, it was all so tight and sore. I found somewhere to hide and I cried. I cried because I'd done it. I cried because my gran would be proud. I cried because I was proud. But more importantly, I cried because I was healing.

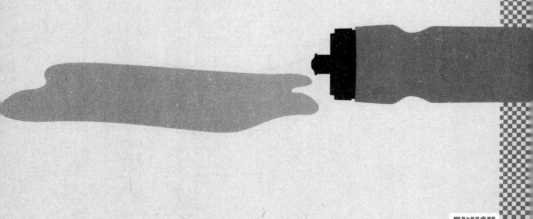

FINISH

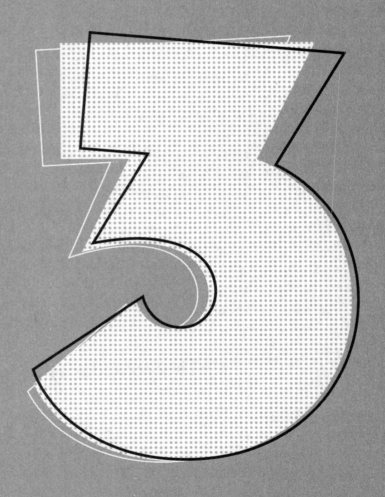

The Mind-Body Connection

The feedback loop

As I began to run more often, I noticed that in the middle of a run my legs would hurt. I would tell them they weren't really hurting, that it was a lie or an elaborate plot to get me to stop and '#stayfat' and I would keep going as if nothing had happened.

Or the opposite would happen and I would be floating along without a care in the world, but for some strange reason I'd have this nagging voice in the back of my head that would say things are going a little *toooo* well, dude . . . You're running too fast, or the pace is too comfortable, something is obviously going to go wrong, ease off. And right after that thought I'd start to really feel the pace. Some negative thoughts like that could impact me negatively. I thought, hmmmmm, maybe there might be some truth to what my mum and gran spent most of my childhood telling me.

Say positive things and positive things will happen. Think and dream big and big things will happen And my favourite, don't say you feel terrible or you will. Of course it's not as simple as that, it's way more complicated. But at its core, for my little brain, it kind of is that simple. This was how I stumbled upon the mind–body connection, when I was already deep into my running journey. It was a like a little loop going from my mind to my body and vice versa.

For those of you that are blissfully unaware of it, the mind–body connection is the notion that our attitude, behaviour, thoughts, feelings and beliefs can positively or negatively affect our bodies. And on the other side of the coin, what we do to our bodies can affect our minds, positively or negatively. What we eat, how much we sleep, and of course how much exercise we do. Think about it. How many times have you been in a bad mood or just not in the best place mentally, and you've gone for a bike ride, to the gym to hit the bag or just for a walk around the block. That exercise, that movement, put a smile on your face, or at least made you feel a little better about yourself and the situation.

On the other hand, when you feel nervous, or excited, you might feel little butterflies in your stomach. Your heart might begin to beat a little quicker and your palms start to get clammy. When you feel confident and happy about something you tend to stand taller, you're more relaxed and far more controlled.

I, as well as many others, often refer to running as the gift that keeps on giving. But in the beginning I didn't know that it was a gift. To me it was like something handed to me that I didn't fully appreciate, not because I was ungrateful but because I had no idea what it did or what it was for. Something that, when it was given, wasn't explained and no one really told me what to expect. They said, open it if you like. So, open it I did. But inside there was this thing with no instructions and no tools to put it together, so I kinda just started.

I was either completely oblivious to all the information, literature and knowledge out there that referenced the wonderful effects of running that live outside the physical side of things, or that information just wasn't as readily available, accessible or acceptable as it is now.

Running was always advertised as something that could add years to your life, making your heart and lungs stronger, burn calories and help with weight management, build strength, increase bone density, or lower blood pressure or cholesterol. At no point did anyone ever say, you know what dude, running can actually make you *feel* better about yourself and your life, too. But then I guess that could also be linked to the fact that in my world no one really spoke openly about mental health and I never really told anyone that there are days that I just don't feel awesome when I rise. Or was it that those that were already very much seasoned runners took for granted the positive effects of running that sat outside the physical? Or maybe they really didn't notice the big smile on their face? It may not happen to everyone, but for some, if you run for long enough, the body releases a range of mood-boosting chemicals. These give you that euphoric feeling that is often referred to as the runner's high.

How amazing is that? How crazy to think that testing yourself physically through running manifests itself in the strengthening of the mind. In the strengthening of your being, the strengthening of that person that lives in all of us, just waiting to jump out and really take on the world. Over the years science has proved that, over time, running can create new brain cells and improve how your brain performs daily. Runs help to improve decision-making skills, higher thinking as well as learning.

You also build patience, grit and determination. Running helps to dampen the brain's response to physical and emotional stress. Exercise increases the levels of endocannabinoids, which flow freely triggering a beautiful euphoric feeling. Endorphins are released, as

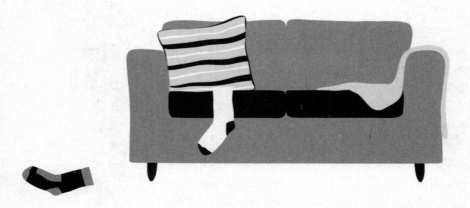

well as serotonin and dopamine which help to enhance your mood, increase your motivation and help improve your memory as your hippocampus (the magical bit in the middle of your brain) grows, enabling you to be more creative and resilient.

When I think back, I realise that the time spent out in the elements chasing my shadow somehow helped make me whole. There's something rewarding about getting up and doing something for nothing. It changes you. It's odd for me to say that, as I have spent so long talking about the benefits of running. My point is no one asks you to run, unless you're an athlete or model, no one pays you to run, and for much of your early running years no one congratulates you for doing it. And to be honest, on most days, especially in the beginning, it's awful. So why would you keep going?

I turned up, no lights, no camera, just action. Just me and the road.

When I first started my back hurt; my stomach, the soles of my feet, my shoulders, my legs, pretty much everywhere hurt. People would feel the need to comment on the big lad trundling down the road looking so uncool . . . but I turned up, no lights, no camera, just action. JUST ME AND THE ROAD.

I noticed it started to create routines, beautiful habits and mental pathways that inevitably helped me be a better version of myself. Prior to running I got up when I had to and never before. Life didn't really excite me – or, should I say, distractions excited me, but life didn't. I had no idea how unhappy I was until I actually started to be happier.

I played football from time to time, tennis, table tennis, dabbled with parkour and occasionally jumped around on a trampoline, but like most people who leave school and don't join a team for team sport's sake I had nothing that really kept me fit or fully motivated. Much of it required dedication, which was something that I'd lost.

I had lost focus, I had stopped caring, about myself and my body. I would pour fizzy drinks down my throat with abandon, gorge on kebabs, devour packs of sweets just because they were in reach during a conversation. I'd chow down on packs of Mr Kipling's finest cakes, but never – not once – did I think about what I was doing to my body, nor did I care. But now, for the first time in a long time, I had a reason to question my relationship with food, with drink, with much of what I had grown accustomed to. Now there was a reason to say NO; now there was a reason to put it down, or better yet a reason to not pick it up at all. Now, just to be clear, I am *not* saying you should NEVER eat fast food, sweets and chocolates, or drink fizzy drinks. What I'm saying is, is there needs to be balance if you want to live your best life.

At the time this logic made no sense. I'm supposed to be fit in order to do this thing that is going to help make me fit. It sounded like hard work, but I was up for it. But I couldn't work out if I was up for it because I was stubborn; because if I said I was going to do something, then by hook or by crook it's going to get done. Or did I continue to pursue what I felt was madness because I just couldn't deal with people thinking they were right all along? And I had *noooo* intention of running?

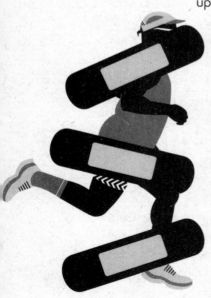

The fact that the act of getting fit actually required me to be fit confused me until I realised that there is a tipping point. A moment you break through and realise you are creating REALLY GOOD HABITS. And as I continued it helped me keep them.

I started to get up a little earlier, which meant I had more time to do the things that I enjoyed. Living in a motivated way

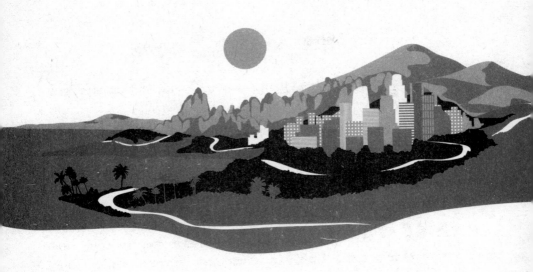

works both for body and mind, and you sometimes need to stage your own intervention.

Running made me realise that with hard work, dedication, sweat, blood and tears you can honestly achieve anything. But it also reiterated the fact that at times IT JUST ISN'T YOUR DAY, and that's okay too.

Running taught me that regardless of how hard you work, no matter how many things go your way, one day the world might just throw you a curve ball and there's nothing you can do about it but react. But here's the thing: the work that you put in when no one is looking is what prepares you for the curve balls, so that when they appear they seem far more manageable. And they look like speed humps not mountains.

I must tell you, in the beginning it felt like all I got was curve balls. All I got was bad weather, injuries, chafing, gastric distress and cramp, while everyone else appeared to be able to run at their leisure. But there's the thing once again. You never actually know what is going through somebody else's head. When you see people float past you on the road you don't know how long they have been running for, when they started, when they will finish or what coping mechanisms they are using to keep that calm, completely unbothered unflustered look on their face – aka The Runner's Poker Face.

At first that Poker Face would annoy the hell out of me. I thought, I'm out here on death's door and these people look like they are having the time of their lives. Until I switched my mindset, I saw them, and simply lied to myself and said *they just started*. They look that calm and collected as they have only been running for a minute, if that long. I would laugh in my head and ask myself if one day I too would be able to look like I had only been running for a minute or so when in fact I'd been out in the cold and wind for well over an hour. (I can now confirm that I have definitely developed my own poker face that I switch on and off from time to time. But when I am really working, really driving and doing my utmost to sit in the little pain cave that I occasionally create, you can see that I am working, you might even hear a grunt from time to time or a scream as I finish a rep and prepare for the next one that starts in 5, 4, 3, 2, 1 – ummmm, NOW . . .)

Comparison can and will be a thief if you are not careful.

I thought a little more about this as time passed, and concluded that regardless of how I looked at it, looking at other runners wasn't helping me. Comparison can and will be a thief if you are not careful. Of course, comparison can inspire too, but in my case it was stealing my joy. I was allowing other people's hard work and dedication to negatively impact me when doing so was, for want of better words, both ludicrous and ridiculous. I was creating my own joy by just being out there and the sooner I understood that, the sooner I could bottle it and sip it whenever I wanted to . . . All would be well. I needed to understand that everyone has different hopes and goals, so why compare myself to anyone else who is either starting out or is further along than me? I shouldn't. And NEITHER SHOULD YOU.

What I had failed to understand is that more often than
not, it was me that was getting in
my own way. It was my own fear that
made me lazy or unwilling to try harder. I
was preventing my own progression. I found that
somehow with running I was able to channel some
of the negative energy that had built up within me
over the years. It was as if every time I put my kicks
on and took to the pavement I was sweating out
some of the baggage I'd carried with me for so
long, the baggage that weighed me down. It
was as if I was stamping on the negativity that
I'd had to navigate, while filling my lungs with
fresh air. That fresh air gave me fresh perspective
on life. That's what fuelled me, that's what helped
to give me the stamina to not just endure life, but
to love it.

It's like the more I ran the more time I had with
myself to process things. Instead of fearing what was to come, I
waited for it.

The more time I spent running, the more time I spent with myself.
And the more time I spent with myself, the more time my brain had
to process everything else that was going on in my world. Of course
I had visions and dreams about the future prior to running but they
were just that, visions and dreams with no real action.

It's unbelievable how the strength that you get from running is
channelled into all areas of your life. Without running, I wouldn't
have the friends that I have, I wouldn't have met my wife, Jules, I
wouldn't have travelled as much as I have and I certainly wouldn't
have been to the places that I have been. Running showed me that
there are people everywhere just like me and I'm not alone. That

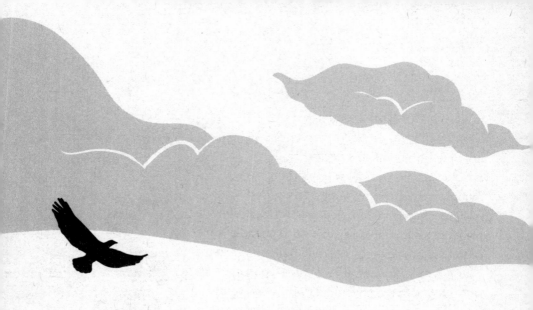

feeling of community is empowering, it makes you feel supported. It puts you in situations that make you think to yourself, under what other circumstances would I be here? And in most instances I can't find one. Through running, both in work and play, I have been blessed with the opportunity to speak with and spend time with some amazing people and athletes.

I remember the day before the London Marathon, many years ago. By then I was the head coach for Nike Run Club in the UK and I was leading a shakeout run for some very lucky Nike Run Club members with three-time winner of the London Marathon, three-time New York Marathon champion and 2002 Chicago Marathon winner Paula Radcliffe MBE. If I haven't sung her praises enough, here's one more for you.

Paula was also previously the fastest female marathoner of all time and held the women's world marathon record for 16 years, from 2003 to 2019, with a time of 2:15:25. Just think about that for a minute. That's 42k in 2 hours 15 minutes 25 seconds. An average of 5 minutes 10 seconds per mile. I remember thinking there was a time when I'd battle to finish a half marathon at that speed. Have I fanboyed enough yet? Should I go on?

Anyhow, we were running along The Mall so people could start

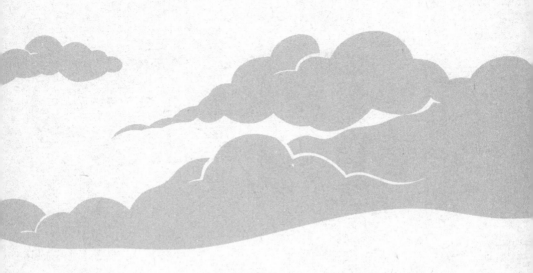

to visualise what the finish would look and feel like and I asked her: 'What do you do when your body hurts and all the glycogen and fuel has gone? What do you tell it? What do you think about? Especially when you are nearing the end and your body is literally eating itself?' She said she calms her mind by staying in the moment and not thinking about how much it hurts or how long she has left. She just thinks about putting one foot in front of the other while counting in her head from 1 to 100. When she hits 100 she either stops counting or, if needs must, she begins the process again.

I smiled – I might have even laughed – as I thought to myself, I am running with the best female British marathon runner of all time and her secret weapon is counting from 1 to 100. My mind was officially blown.

We may not all run at the highest level or be record holders but we can certainly take inspiration from this. The body does what the mind tells it to. And when you don't know what to tell your body to do, just fool it into believing that everything is okay . . . Until it's not, but hopefully you'll have got where you're going by then. It might sound cheesy, but you, my friend, are the master of your own destiny. So, as we say trackside, OWN IT.

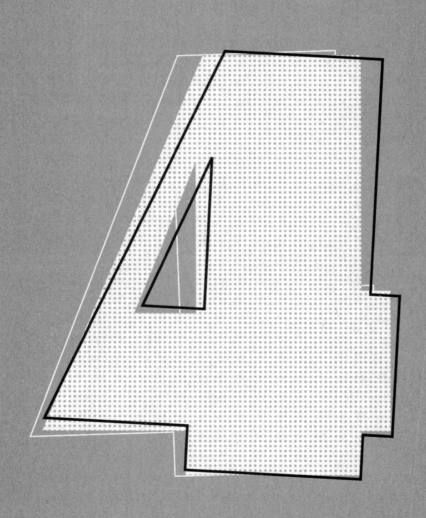

Pick Up the Pace

How to get better

People often ask me, once you started running, at what point did you decide that you wanted to get better? At what point did you want to improve and fine tune the engine that you'd started to build?

For months I just focused on running a little bit further and a little bit longer each time, and aimed to get to a point where I didn't feel like every time I hit the road I'd expire there and then. And it worked; I found a steady rhythm, my base pace, and I could run without feeling and looking like a hungover bear. But then . . . I got the bug and wanted to get more serious. I could see my progression, I could see that I was getting better, accomplishing something that I had previously deemed improbable, if not impossible. Thinking about it now it seems crazy that I wanted to get out there and do more – it hurt. But I was spurred on by all of this being measurable. I could clearly see my progress and it felt good.

I liked that my body was starting to do things that it couldn't do before, and deep, deep down, whatever light was flickering inside me seemed to get brighter as I moved. Running gave me the confidence to want to try more. Outside of that it also seemed like the right thing to do, it was a natural progression. Whatever I was doing was making me feel better, when I didn't know a better existed.

> **Whatever I was doing was making me feel better, when I didn't know a better existed.**

When the time comes for you to pick it up a little, ask yourself, why am I doing this? There's no right answer, just your answer, your truth. For me it was searching for something that I didn't know I needed: clarity on who I am. I view my brain like a white table, a bit like an office table, and someone has dumped boxes of photos on the table.

It's a mess, and running helps me put all those pictures in pretty little piles and patterns that help me see the world the way I need to see it, to live in it with a smile on my face and love in my heart. This is what the runs tap for me. I also picked it up because I thought another goal would help motivate me to keep running. I wanted to run so I could eat more, I wanted to run so I had something to do, it gave me a passion outside of work. It gave me a passport to explore, something to share, an opportunity to go to places I would never have gone.

The first thing I will say is that getting better requires commitment and patience. You aren't going to get better overnight. It takes time, small incremental steps and half steps – and setbacks. If you sign up to get better and always bear those few things in mind, your magical journey will continue to make you smile.

In the early days it's possible that you'll see improvements fairly quickly. In comparison, when you have been running for a lot longer, the better you get the fewer areas there are for you to improve in, while the things that you change can have less of an impact.

The following suggestions are things you can consider doing once you've decided you want to step it up, things to help you progress and grow as a runner. Now when I say grow as a runner I don't just mean getting faster, I mean getting stronger, being more mobile, more flexible, having a better understanding of your body and, of course, your mind. How will your body recover from the mileage in races and in training? What do you have to do more of or less of to reach your goals? These are questions we should all ask ourselves, and the suggestions below can help you get there.

1

Enter a race

If you're just starting your running journey, or even if you've been running for a while, a great way to start getting better is to pick a challenge that you can commit to. Just having something in the diary, something to train for, can give you a little extra focus, something to gear your training towards. On days when you might not want to head out for a run, it provides another reason to get out the door. Of course, your health and the possibility of living a longer life are reasons enough! But why not have more of an incentive? I'll touch more on that in Chapter 6, 'Set Goals'.

Just know that you can start slow, run any distance from a mile to hundreds of miles, solo or as a team, free or paid for, on roads, beaches and through forests. If you're wondering how you go about finding these races, then Google or any kind of search engine is your friend. You can cast the Net as broadly or as narrowly as you like. As narrow as '5k running races near me' or as broad as 'best running races in the world' of any distance. Ask and you shall find. There are many websites dedicated to finding races dependent on what country you're in. But I tend to use the Runner's World website or Active.com. Or I will search for the best 5k, 10k, half marathon, marathon or relay races, then go directly to the race's website and enter there.

Now some of you might want to know if there are any races that cater specifically for beginners. I'd say there aren't as all are very welcoming. When entering, though, check to see if there's a qualifying time for a race, or what the cut-off time is, if there is one, for a particular distance. My advice is always when you first start running, begin with a small, small race such as a local 5k or mile race so you can get used to running with other people, seeing and feeling what the whole experience is like; it can be a little daunting being surrounded by lots of other runners. As you get more comfortable and gain experience, increase the distance and the size of the race. If your goal is to do a marathon, go slowly, build: 5k, 10k, half marathon, marathon. But when you do pick your first marathon, PICK A BIG ONE. Smaller races are great, but if you're going to do ONE, you want the streets lined with people screaming and shouting your name as that will give you such a big energy boost. (See Chapter 8: 'Time for an Adventure', for more info on races.)

To be honest, even after I had run two or three marathons, a bunch of half marathons and smaller races, I said to myself, dude, you may have these races under your belt, but you still have no idea what you're doing, do you? What are you going to do about it? There was still so much left for me to do both mentally and physically if I wanted to grow as a runner.

Right then, my goal was to simply finish a marathon, either in a time that I was happy with, or feeling proud in another way that had nothing to do with time but was to do with my attitude, how I applied what I'd learnt about running to the run itself. If I could do that, I'd be happy.

Not long after running the New York Marathon I made that decision; I knew I needed more help, and I went to find it.

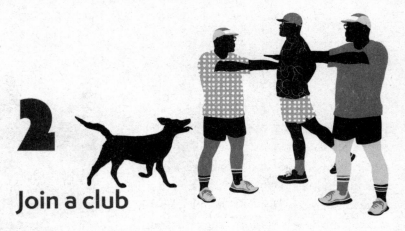

2

Join a club

Running clubs are great in a number of ways. They give you a reason to get out there and run on days when you may not feel like running alone, or running at all. They are great for camaraderie, a place for you to feel at home like you are part of a family with a shared love. They are filled with tons of people who can give you advice, share knowledge, personal experiences, hacks and more. And don't forget they are great places to simply meet other runners who you can spend time with, run, share the road, and have a lot of fun with.

I joined Dulwich Runners running club and started putting in work with them on the track and road. Many of the magical journeys that I have been on around the world have involved spending hours pounding the pavements with people who were once strangers.

The same strangers helped me lose a lot of weight, even though they knew that wasn't why I was there. One day one of the runners said that they admired my commitment, but if I really wanted to maximise my chances of becoming a better runner I should work on shifting the bags of sugar that I had strapped to my waist. Some might say she overstepped some boundaries by commenting on my weight or appearance, *but* . . . I looked at her and couldn't even be mad, as she wasn't rude, she didn't put me down or say it to upset me, she was giving me facts. (See Chapter 8 for more on run clubs.)

That was one of the many kicks up the behind I needed to up the ante a little bit and shift some weight. It was the first time I really ventured into exploring nutrition of any kind.

3

Drop some weight

It was good advice for me and I took it on board. That advice may not have been for everyone, but right then it was what I needed. I *was* overweight. I had to be honest with myself. At the time my weight was holding me back and I wasn't happy. I wasn't big boned, dense, thick or too muscly, I was fat. And I'm not going to pretend I wasn't. Things probably would have been different if I had developed enough muscle to carry all the weight around, but I hadn't.

Remember, this advice is NOT for everyone. It is for those of you that need to see it. Regardless of what your weight is, you are amazing, you are loved and you are beautiful. I am telling you about what I needed to do to get where I was going. It may not apply to you, because your weight isn't holding you back. But if you think it is, give this section a read. I'm saying this as I don't want people to think that in order to run or be a runner you have to be a certain weight or look a certain way. That is not the case!

If you feel like making a change to your weight, it could be helpful to you, too. I wanted to lose weight because back then I thought it was a simple maths problem: lighter = faster. And to be lighter I needed to lose weight. To lose weight I just needed to burn more calories than I consumed and create a calorie deficit. It turned out to be a great entry point to gaining a better understanding of nutrition as a whole and how it fuelled my body.

I know now that it's a little more complicated than simply EAT LESS, BURN MORE. There's a lot of literature out there about individual body make-up and how weight loss can be accomplished – and whether that's the right thing for you to aim for. But at the time it was all I knew, and even though I thought I'd never be someone who counted calories I found it helped me. For the first time I had a reason to track what I was eating.

It's a little more complicated than simply eat less, burn more.

I went online and read up about the Resting (or Basal) Metabolic Rate (RMR or BMR) — that's the number of calories needed to keep your body working when it's doing nothing all day; for example, if you just woke up and didn't move, just lay there taking breaths. The RMR indicates how many calories you would need a day to do that. And that number depends on a bunch of things like age, weight, gender and how active you are.

At the time I still weighed well over 100kg, which meant my Resting Metabolic Rate was around 2,200 calories, so that's what I needed just to survive.

If you want to try working yours out you can either use the Web, an app or do the maths yourself. You just need a calculator and your notes, or if you're old school, a pen and a pad. You can use the Harris–Benedict Equation below, a formula that needs your age, weight and height. It's not an exact science, and it may not be entirely accurate for certain people because it doesn't distinguish between fat and muscle in body mass. But at the time, for my purposes, it was close enough:

HARRIS–BENEDICT EQUATION

Men	BMR = 88.362 + (13.397 x weight in kg) + (−.799 x height in cm) - (5.677 x age in years)
Women	BMR = 447.593 + (9.247 x weight in kg) + (−.098 x height in cm) - (4.330 x age in years)

After a little more research and straight-up honesty with myself I found out that if I wanted to lose 30lb (13.6kg) in weight in a healthy way, a way that I could manage and maintain, I should work on dropping somewhere between 1lb (0.45kg) and 2lb (0.9kg) a week.

I surprised myself and was accidentally an early over-achiever, as for the first four to eight weeks of taking my eating seriously I dropped between 1kg and 2kg a week. Then after the first 8kg fell off, things started to get a little harder. It was about being smart and understanding that this wasn't some quick painful fad diet that was going to leave me feeling hungry and fatigued. This was a lifestyle change that I planned to stick with. It wasn't about starving myself, it was about finding the balance between being able to enjoy eating the things I wanted to or liked, and doing so in moderation. The moment I realised that I could have a cookie, just not ten in one sitting and at midnight, I started to transform.

There are lots of good sources out there that recommend losing weight gradually if you decide to do it. Honestly, fad diets don't work! If you want to lose weight — for health, to improve your running performance, or otherwise — do it healthily and slowly. You'll feel better for it, and it's easier to stick to as long as you are honest with yourself. Now, can I repeat, I am not saying that as a runner you *need* to lose weight, I am saying when I started to run, *I* for sure needed to lose weight. Dropping weight made running easier for me and I was less prone to injury. It may not be the case for you. But for me, it needed to go.

It's a simple maths problem. Imagine yourself running at your current weight. Now imagine nothing else changing except I hand you two 5kg dumbbells to run with or give you a 10kg weight vest to run in. Is it going to be easier or harder to run with the weights? *That* was essentially my problem. I needed to take the weighted vest off and drop the dumbbells.

4

Look at what you eat

Now the reason I'm telling you all this is at that point in time I wasn't simply counting calories. I was starting to take ownership of my health, beginning to get a better understanding of what my body was doing, and of what I was doing to my body with what I was putting in it. It was then that I understood that to get better I needed to also think about what I did before, during and after the run. Think about it this way: how are you supposed to build the house of your dreams without the right materials?

At the time I loved Bakewell tarts. A Bakewell tart contains around 200 calories and in order to burn 200 calories I worked out I needed to bike for 30 minutes at 10mph, jog for 25 minutes or walk briskly for 45 minutes. That put it all into perspective and from then on I looked at that Bakewell tart in tandem with what I would I have to put my body through to eat it. I started making food decisions based on that.

This is what worked for me, this was my motivator, but it might not work for you. Take an honest look at what and how you eat and ask yourself this question: are there any tweaks that could help you improve as a runner? I'm not talking about taking a deep dive into nutrition, I'm talking about quick wins. We know that drinking a gallon of Coke and eating a ton of cake, burgers and sweets isn't smart. Yet many of us still do it, so the next time you're thinking about the sneaky snacks and fast foods say, 'Is this conducive to my running journey and helping me get better?' Even if you still continue, at least you're aware and have had the conversation.

I said to myself, dude . . . of course you are overweight, you eat six Bakewell tarts at a time.

As for me, of course I continued to treat myself occasionally, but I stopped eating six Bakewell tarts at a time. I said to myself, dude . . . of course you are overweight, you eat six Bakewell tarts at a time. That's 1,200 calories of trash in one sitting, *over half* of what you should be eating in a day. So instead of six I'd have one and not feel guilty about it.

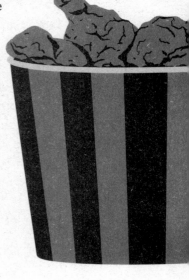

I'm not for one minute saying the weight just fell off, but I realised how much trash I had been eating and how much easier it was to run – or simply carry my body – when I had less of a body to carry around.

Getting better is all about realising the little things you can do to help you improve as a runner. After working out what wasn't great for me to be eating, I dug into what I could eat instead to help fuel my runs. I looked for advice everywhere, and the more I read the more I had *aha* moments. Back then I spent a lot of time on the Runner's World website, geeking out on articles as well as reading the magazine. I hit up *Athletics Weekly* and *Men's Health*, then read books like *What I Talk About When I Talk About Running* by Haruki Murakami, *Born to Run* by Christopher McDougall, *Eat and Run* by Scott Jurek and *Ultra Marathon Man* by Dean Karnazes.

I took something different from each of these books, which helped me to form my feelings about what kind of runner I might be. I not only spent time with my head in these books but I also trawled the Internet, watched videos on YouTube and Google, or downloaded stuff and watched it on RealPlayer. I also went to libraries and looked for anything that made running sound remotely like fun, while combining it with a sprinkling of 'Wow, these people are wild'. I realised that I needed to feel a little bit of a wow factor when I read about these people. They needed to seem superhuman but at the same time normal. It inspired me to think that a normal person could do what they did, so me being a normal person too ... encouraged me to believe I could do my bit.

I looked for advice everywhere, and the more I read the more I had aha moments.

When it comes to food and what you can eat to run well, there is far too much to share here, but I came away with a few key ideas I still stick to today. I aim to eat healthily in a way that gives me enough energy for my runs and makes me feel good too. Here are those ideas.

5

Carbo load *only* when you need to

The first thing I realised was that the reason I had put on so much weight *after* I first started running was because I felt that I had to carbo load every time I stepped out the house lol. Of course, many people put on weight during marathon training due to an increase in fuelling, but I had been excessive and put on *waaaaaay* too much.

Now, just in case you didn't know what carbo loading is, it means consuming a lot more carbs than you would normally to help increase the amount of energy you have stored in your body as glycogen. Glycogen is a source of fuel that your body taps into to help keep you running. Carbo loading is usually helpful before a race or a long run, when you know you'll need loads of energy to get to the finish. In the beginning I was eating a bowl of pasta the size of my head just to run to the bottom of the road and back. I now know I *didn't have to do that*.

As long as I was eating a balanced diet consisting of the right amount of carbs, proteins and fats, I only really needed to carbo load if I planned on exercising for more than 90 minutes. All the energy or glycogen that I needed to do less than that was already stored in my body (muscles, liver, red blood cells and kidneys), so all the other stuff I was eating was just making me heavier. Sure, it would keep me warm in the winter, but it wasn't what I needed in order to run.

Complex carbs versus simple carbs

Carbs are your friend! You can consume simple carbs or complex carbs. Both have a role to play when running.

Complex carbs help you prepare for and recover from runs and races. They build up and store glycogen to provide longer lasting energy, or to help with recovery from workouts and races. They take longer to burn through leaving you fuller for longer, providing energy at a slower rate. Great complex carbs are those that are high in starch like wholegrain bread, cereal and pasta, but if you really want to go in on the complex carbs try some quinoa (pronounced *keen*-wah) or buckwheat.

Don't overdo it. Remember, BALANCED.

They are great alternatives to pasta and rice, and are available from normal supermarkets. Both are rich in fibre and protein so you feel fuller longer after eating them, and runners love them — I like to include them in my meals every week. (I mean who ever thought I'd say the word BUCKWHEAT, let alone know what it was, and eat it and then tell you about it?)

If you want easily accessible, fairly instant energy, go for simple carbs and sugars. They give you a quick energy boost that also passes quickly. They can be found in things like milk, fruit, sugar, corn syrup, fruit juice concentrate and sports drinks and gels.

Energy gels are carbohydrate gels that provide energy for exercise and help promote recovery. They come in little packets that you can fit in your pockets or a little running belt and they can be found in specialist running, trail or cycling shops, as well as most supermarkets in the 'healthy' section. But each place varies with regards to which brands they carry. Maurten tends to be the go-to brand for record breakers, but don't quote me lol. I personally use them, also SIS and Cliff. There's also torq, GU Energy, Lucozade – *sooooo* many.

I would suggest including complex carbs in your weekly balanced diet and when you've got a long run or race. Have them as part of your breakfast, lunch and dinner, especially in the days leading up to a race. But don't overdo it. Remember, BALANCED.

The simple carbs and sugars are used for a boost of energy before your run or race, or during a run or race. When I race, especially in a half marathon or marathon, I tend to have a gel or another simple carb or sugar every 30 minutes. It's also true that if I'm just going out for a quick 30-minute run I will take on some instant energy to get me going.

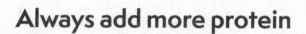

Always add more protein

Rumour has it that protein is an edible upgrade for your legs – it helps to build muscle as well as repair all the micro tears you make in your muscles during exercise. So I've found ways to add more protein to my meals. Protein-rich foods include eggs, chicken, milk, shellfish, lean beef, fish and turkey to name but a few. If meat, fish and dairy products are not for you, protein can also be found in almonds, lentils, quinoa, peanuts and peanut butter.

7

Eat real food

Ultimately, eating well as a runner boils down to eating healthily. If you consider your body to be like a car, it's just about throwing some stuff out so the vehicle is lighter and changing the fuel you put in so it runs more efficiently. This amounts to consuming less junk food and more fruit, veg and unprocessed ingredients. I didn't follow any strict eating plan, I just tried to eat 'well' most of the time, and to be honest it's still what I aim for. It gets easier, but it's never *easy*. It will always be a work in progress, and there's nothing wrong with that.

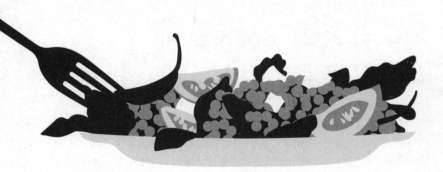

8

Recovery and sleep

Next up an even bigger surprise – SLEEP. I know when some of you read the chapter title 'Pick Up the Pace' you thought that it was all going to be about reps and sets and speed and workouts and all the other magical things that get our attention, but actually it's the things that don't get the headlines that can really help us. So here is the secret all runners know: SLEEP IS YOUR SECRET WEAPON. SLEEP IS LIKE HITTING THE BACKUP AND REBOOT BUTTON EVERY NIGHT.

As you sleep, your body is literally HEALING ITSELF. Working its little butt off repairing itself so you can wake up feeling stronger and healthier. Hormones are released that promote and encourage tissue growth. This helps cuts and bruises to heal faster as well as working on healing sore or damaged muscles.

The National Sleep Foundation advises that healthy adults need between seven and nine hours of sleep per night. And not getting that *can* negatively impact your immune system. But getting enough sleep can *positively* impact your immune system. I used to find that I'd slip into a cycle. I wouldn't get enough sleep, then I'd spend all day eating trash to give me energy quickly because I was tired. That trash wasn't good for my body, so I would put on more weight. So my advice to you is get as much sleep as you can.

Treat your body a little better and it will treat you better.

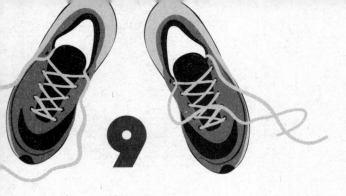

Take the time and space you need

In the beginning I would think that taking so long to ready myself for the road was an act of fear, delaying the inevitable, when in actual fact I was prolonging the ritual. I was making time, finding space in a busy world to BREATHE, to experience that breath, to get my mind right. Then, for whatever reason, I would put thumping music on that didn't help me to explore what I'd just found – it did more to drown it out.

But now, now I get it. Now I understand why I moved so slowly. Slowly gathering my things, thinking about my run, thinking about what route I'll take, thinking about what the weather is like, the temperature, I start to consider how the ground is going to feel, and whether or not that will change during this new mission. My eyes start to wander but always come back to the centre. I always click my back and neck while rolling my shoulders, thinking, is this going to be a good run? Or will I be tested? One thing I do know is that, regardless of what kind of a run it is, it's the run I'm supposed to have, so I embrace it.

This is ALL PART OF GETTING BETTER. Giving myself the time and the space that I need to really immerse myself in what I'm doing. Kind of like a moving meditation.

When I'm at home I always sit on the same step and look at the same place on the same patch of floor and say 'thank you'. Without this personal ritual I know my mind would be a little darker, a little less light. I smile at the thought of all this light, then grab my kicks and lace up. It's only really then that I start to move any quicker. I know it's time for the switch, as I get my body and my mind into a different gear.

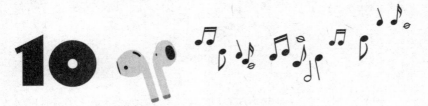

10

Music? First, listen to your body

In the beginning, when it came down to music, my attitude was simple: play music that inspired me to move, play music to get me hyped and through my run. But, more importantly, play music to drown out the noise of my suffering. That THUD THUD THUD, the sound of my feet hitting the floor in such an inelegant manner. The sound of me gasping for air, panting when I had only been running for a few minutes. I needed to play loud music so I didn't feel embarrassed. I mean how sad is that? The problem is that as I never listened to myself, I never actually knew how I sounded. I just presumed.

I remember loading up my iPod with nothing but drum and bass and jungle music and just going for it. It wasn't until I clocked myself in the reflection of a parked car that I realised how ridiculous I looked with my flailing arms and weird gait. I didn't look like the Olympian that I thought I did, nor did I feel like one.

My boss Eugene Minogue and I were at a function in South London somewhere when we had the privilege of meeting the Olympic Gold medallist Sally Gunnell. We got to talking, and Eugene and I let her know that he was in fact a trained gymnast and I was an endurance athlete. The joke of it was neither of us looked like what we had just described. When she'd realised we were indeed deadly serious I said I planned to run my first marathon soon and I asked if she had any

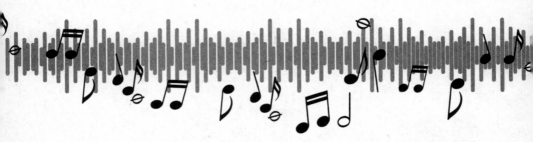

advice. She said yes and asked such a simple question – she asked if I listened to music. I said yes, thinking she was planning on exchanging playlists, and I mentally lined up some banging tunes for her, but what she actually said sticks with me till this day.

She said 'Stop, *don't* listen to music; how are you supposed to listen to your body?'

At the time I didn't realise what a gem she had just given me, I just thought, *ahhhhhh*, okay, our gold medallist here reckons drum and bass isn't going to get me a gold medal and I should listen. So I *stopped*.

The next time I went out for a run, I went out with no music, just the sound of suffering. And within a few metres I realised good old Sally Gunnell was right — so if you're reading or listening, Sally, thank you for taking the time.

Now just because she was right, doesn't mean I was happy, as now I could hear everything; I sounded like a steam train, just chugging along. But it wasn't the sound of my feet hitting the floor that was deafening, it was the sound of silence. The problem with silence is you actually have to listen to yourself. You have to process things that you have hidden, things you've shut off or filed away, things you've compartmentalised and said, 'That's TRAUMA', leave that where it is. What's worse than things you know you are running from? Things you didn't even know were there.

Of course, now I was no longer chasing the beat or inspiration from the DnB bpm that had kept me raving all night long all those

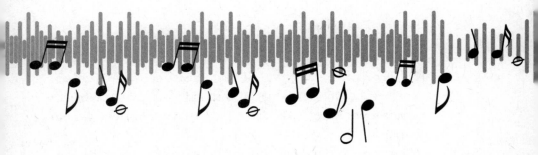

years ago, I could also hear my body and I was hearing things I didn't like. But hearing them allowed me to work on them.

After listening a while I noticed that my pace slowed, my breathing was far more regulated, and I started to care less about how fast I was going and more about how I felt and what I could see. After that first run without music I didn't run to music for a long while.

Now when I coach, and people ask what my thoughts are on music, my response is always, as with many things, that music has both a time and place, especially in the running space. I tell people that music is a great tool for inspiration and motivation. But it's not something that we should become solely dependent on. We live in a world of 'what ifs', so I ask you this: what if your battery died mid race? Or at the beginning of a race? How would you feel? Could you still go on? If you could, then you are already one step ahead of where I was. If you couldn't, this is a great opportunity to start to work towards that freedom.

Just to be really clear here, I *love* music, and I get to choose great running playlists for runners as a part of my full-time job with Apple Fitness+. Coach Cory is not saying never listen to music when you run. I'm saying music is a gift, it's inspirational, motivational and a beautiful tool that can and should be used to help propel you to your goals. *But* if you have never

> **I was hearing things I didn't like. But hearing them allowed me to work on them.**

unplugged and listened to yourself move, listened to yourself run, listened to the way you land, listened to your body — LISTENED TO YOU — you are doing yourself a disservice and missing out on something beautiful. And that is the sound of suffering combined with the sound of you taking flight and floating along. Your version of flying.

One of the most beautiful sounds I have ever heard is 20-plus people running together, footstrike and breathing all in unison . . . No one talking, just working, driving onward to a place some-where far away. It's like a symphony, all are there sharing this experience, all battling to stay in that moment, that running nirvana.

My suggestion is, just like training, to always mix your running up. Do some runs with music and some runs without and if you can help it, try and do the first part of your runs without music so you and your body can find its own natural rhythm. That way you're not chasing the rhythm of the track.

When you do use music, a great way to get better is to build a playlist that ties in with your workout — and if you are a geek like me or an up-and-coming DJ you can build out your playlist so it ebbs and flows with your intensity or pace. If you know you start to get tired, say, at around 20 minutes, make sure you put one of your favourite songs at the 20-minute mark to give you a little boost or take your mind off the time.

A disclaimer: remember, these are just my learnings, based on my experiences. If the thought of running without music terri-fies you and without it you just wouldn't run *at all*, then IGNORE EVERYTHING YOU JUST READ and keep making those playlists that work for you. The end goal is simply to run.

Once you are in a place where you know your body, play your power song to your heart's content. When it's time, and it feels right, I too can be found floating along, singing and humming, sometimes sprinting and grimacing, but always taken on a journey by the music.

What's interesting is when I row or cycle or do any other kind of killer cardio I am straight in on the tunes as that really helps me get in the zone. But not with running – like I said, there's a time and place.

11

Podcasts, fitness apps and trackers

If music isn't your thing try listening to podcasts or audio books, or even listen to me or some of the other coaches on Apple's Fitness+ Time to Run or the Nike Run Club app.

Find what works for you. For me, still, the greatest tool at your disposal is your mind, but admittedly there are times when the mind needs a little something extra. There are so many options to help enhance your run.

Podcasts and audiobooks are great. They not only take your mind off the running but they can also help to boost your productivity. Have you ever wanted to read a book and said *ahhhh*, I just don't have the time? Or you might have a book on the go, but you want a change. Well, why not download an audiobook and listen while you run? WIN-WIN. You could listen to this book when you're running, or you could listen to something completely different.

The same thing applies to podcasts. There are so many different genres covering news, comedy, society and culture, fashion,

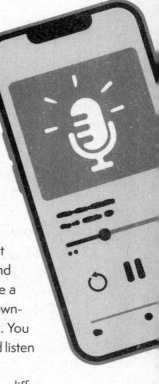

business, true crime, science, TV and film, religion, sport, health and fitness, history, music, fiction, and on and on. You have a lot of options to listen, learn and take your mind off the run. Listening to podcasts can also give you extra motivation to do other things outside of your run. It might pique your interest in a new hobby, or you could learn something about running or nutrition or another type of training to complement your running journey.

This leads beautifully into why having a coach in your ear offering running tips and tricks and giving you motivation can be so beneficial, especially if you're unable to hire a personal trainer or running coach. Better yet, if you are fortunate enough to have a coach already, you can use your in-ear coach to supplement the pre-planned sessions that your original coach gave you. An example of this would be, your coach says go run 10k easy. They've given you your plan, told you what to do, you just want or need a little extra motivation. I say this as I know from personal experience nothing beats a friendly voice in your ear telling you, 'You are awesome,' telling you to keep digging and telling you you've only got one mile, lap or hill left to go. It takes out the guesswork and it means that you can concentrate on getting out there and being your best badass self.

Do I use them? Of course I do. I don't listen to my own guided runs, that would be a little bit weird lol . . . But I listen to my friends and I listen to other coaches. I find them to be more useful for shorter runs between 1 mile and 10k, or for intervals, track workouts or fartlek training when I really, really need a push (see Chapter 5), while I listen to audiobooks, podcasts and Time To Walk on longer runs.

12

Find your breath

When you allow yourself to listen to your body, the first thing you'll hear is your breath. This is a brilliant opportunity to think about your breathing and how much what you hear correlates to the amount of effort that you are putting in.

I learnt a lot about this in the early days from my first proper running coach, Barbara Brunner (known to everyone as Coach Babs). One day she put me on the treadmill, and after a decent enough warm-up she banged the incline and speed up and said, 'Run.' Then she put the speed up some more and said, 'Keep running!' until I was nearly out of breath lol. She said, 'This, Cory, this is what we must work on.' I said, 'What? Me looking like a hot mess?' She said, 'No, your

At that moment it clicked in my head. I must control everything with the rhythm of my breath.

form falls apart when you are tested. Your arms are flailing around, your breathing is really off, it's just not all together.' I said, 'So, not the right rhythm?' She said, 'Exactly.'

At that moment it clicked in my head. I must control everything with the rhythm of my breath because without oxygen I can only do things for a short period of time. So I must find a way. She put me back on the treadmill and said, 'RUN, but now you control the pace on the treadmill and find a pattern so that your breathing is synced in unity with your arm drive and your footstrike. It doesn't matter what the rhythm is as long as it's consistent. If it changes you will know if it's right for you or wrong for you.'

First, I started breathing through my nose so it was controlled, but when I increased my pace I switched to breathing through my mouth and my mouth was wide open. The reason I switched was simple; if you're really, really thirsty and someone hands you a pint glass full of water, do you grab a straw and sip slowly or do you put the glass to your mouth and neck it? I personally neck it, and that's how I looked at breathing. The pretty controlled way through my nose was the straw and necking it was breathing with my mouth wide open.

I started off with a simple rhythm, and found that just being more aware of my breathing brought this feeling of calm to my body and instead of breathing into my chest I was breathing deep into my diaphragm. The rhythm was 2:2 or 3:3 when I first started, which meant I'd inhale for two or three footstrikes then exhale for two or three footstrikes. But then we worked on trying to switch it up so that I wasn't always breathing out when landing on the same foot. I'd try and breathe in for three and breathe out for two. Meanwhile my arm drive was following exactly what my legs were doing. After weeks of doing sessions on the treadmill she said, 'Let's take it to the road.'

We went out on the canal path, Coach Babs on a bike cycling beside me with a loudhailer, monitoring my running and breathing. We'd do short intervals to see that I was doing it all correctly. We found that I was slipping back into 2:2 or 3:3 when I started to get tired, but I was still in control and no longer panicking. Whatever we were doing was working. When I start coaching people nowadays, it's one of the first things we discuss, finding calm by finding your breath, regardless of how fast you're going or where you're running. Your breath is always there.

So how does that help all your runs? It helps to inform you how the breathing should feel, it gives you a way of pressing a reset button and bringing calm to yourself, like a moving meditation.

Find calm by finding your breath, regardless of how fast you're going or where you're running.

On an easy run, it should feel like you could run for forever and a day. It's easy for you to breathe, it's comfortable and you feel completely in control and can have a proper conversation with no trouble at all. If you're running with friends, do just that, talk to them about your day and let them do the same. If you are running by yourself, try singing your favourite song, or tell yourself repeatedly how amazing you are for getting out there and running.

If we were to rate this effort it should feel like a 3 to 4 out of 10, 1 being strolling on the beach and 10 being running flat out from a dinosaur for fear of being eaten.

On a medium or moderate-paced run your breathing should be a little heavier but not laboured. It should still be fairly comfortable but you might feel it starting to become a little more challenging. You will still be able to hold a conversation, but that conversation is now a lot shorter as you have started to choose your words a little more wisely to save air.

If we were to rate this effort it should feel like a 5 to 6 out of 10. This is around the effort that you are looking for if you are new to running and you are taking on a half marathon or marathon.

On a hard run your pace will be uncomfortable but manageable for a certain amount of time, and you can just about manage to pull a very short sentence together. But you are not happy that someone has asked you to speak.

If we were to rate this effort it should feel like a 7 to 8 out of 10. With training this is around the level of effort that you are looking for, for a 5k or 10k.

I had been running for a few years when I started to try and attack some of the races that I was entering, but in every race I seemed to get caught up in a pack that I had no business being in. Due to my lack of experience and not fully understanding my body or what it was capable of I'd be *gasssssed* out before we even hit halfway. It wasn't until I really started to pay attention to my breathing that I began to get it right. I knew I had the endurance to run the pace, I just got very nervous and made silly mistakes like letting adrenalin take over from my beautifully crafted race plan. I just couldn't go out *hard* at the pace that I was trying to, as my heart and lungs just *screamed* NOOOOOOO, DON'T DO IT at me. I discovered that finding my breath really helped me to set out at the right pace. I made a habit of talking to someone else, or to myself, for the first few minutes or miles of a race while I was settling into my rhythm. I knew that if I could speak comfortably I was okay, while if I couldn't I needed to slow down.

As time passed I started to get used to what my body did at certain paces simply based on my breathing, and the fitter I got the faster I could run and still manage to speak comfortably. Getting better has so much to do with getting to know your body. So do just that. Become friends.

13

Get a coach

My next piece of advice on getting better is to invest time, money and resources into someone that knows more than you, someone that you can build trust with, someone who isn't just there to take your money. Someone who cares about you, about running and the culture of running. Don't get me wrong, I promise to give you all the wisdom I have to impart in this book, and hopefully this will get you a long way, but if you want to take things more seriously and push it to the next level, even if that level is from beginner to non-beginner, there is nothing in this world that beats one-on-one coaching, even if it's just one or two sessions. Deciding to call upon someone with experience to hold my hand was honestly one of the best decisions I made about running and life. I know it's costly and it's a big ask, but if you can, you won't regret it.

I have found that the best way to find a good running coach is with receipts. And when I say with receipts I mean from other people who have benefited from a particular good coach so they recommend them to you. Or someone that comes recommended by a community; even though you don't know anyone personally who has been coached by them, you can see or speak to people who have. They have receipts . . . testimonials, whether written or verbal, saying how wonderful they are. You can find these receipts on coaches' websites, social media and elsewhere. *But* just because they were or are a good coach to someone else it doesn't mean that they are going to be a good coach to you. I say this because a good coach isn't simply someone who knows what workout you should be doing, how fast you should be running or what you should be lifting. A good coach gets to know you and starts to understand what motivates *you*, how far to push *you* (or not). A good coach understands what you need to be your best self, and building that bond takes time. Of course, a personal trainer could help you hit those running goals too, but they may miss out on some of the nuances of running that I have grown to appreciate.

A good coach gets to know you and starts to understand what motivates you.

I was put onto Barbara Brunner by Charlie Dark at RunDemCrew (more about them in Chapter 9). She was already coaching and treating a few of the other runners. I had been coached before but always as part of a group. Originally, I went to see her because I kept getting injured and I was told that she could help to fix me. I wasn't expecting what I encountered.

We arranged an appointment at her studio in Shoreditch. I explained that I had run a few marathons, but they didn't go to plan, and I wanted her help preventing injuries so I could spend more time running. This was five or six years after I started running. She laughed and made a quip about not getting injured, then told me to jump on the treadmill and just run for a little bit at a pace that I was comfortable at. I ran for a little while, then she told me to jump off and gave me her verdict.

'I can see why you may get injured so frequently and I can see where we can improve your running. You run like a cross between a footballer or boxer and a little sloth.'

In that moment I could have done one of two things: either be really offended or find out what she meant. I went for the latter. I said, 'Sloths don't run.' She said, 'Exactly.'

She explained there was far too much movement from my trunk, far too much rotation, I was carrying my arms too high and I might not be wearing the best footwear for my style of running. She could see I had poor mobility and range of motion, my body was too tight and it was holding me back. She said my breathing was off, I had no power in my glutes, my hamstrings were tight and I had a lot of tension *everywhere*.

'There's nothing wrong with running like a footballer if you're playing football, but if you're not chasing a ball there's a more efficient way to run, especially if you are going to be running for hours.'

She changed my life with those few words. I wasn't offended or put off by them. I took them from the place that she intended them to come from, and that place was one of love. I always felt supported by Babs; there was A LOT OF WORK TO DO and she showed her respect by letting me know that from the jump. She didn't mince words or pander to my ego, she just needed to know that I was in, and so she was all in too.

Running coaches start with a running MOT, not too dissimilar to one that a car gets, checking in on all the injuries that you have or had, your current little niggles and future goals, before putting a plan in place. It helped me learn even more about running and my body and how much little things can impact your run. Your coach will take a 360-degree view of what you need to improve in all areas and tell you what to target and how, things that would take longer to work out on your own.

Babs coached me one on one for years, and even though we now live in different countries and different time zones she is still the first person I call if my body goes *ping* and needs to be sewn back together. So if you do go and search for a coach, make sure you are interviewing them and they are interviewing you, as that bond is special and important. You are essentially putting your body in their hands.

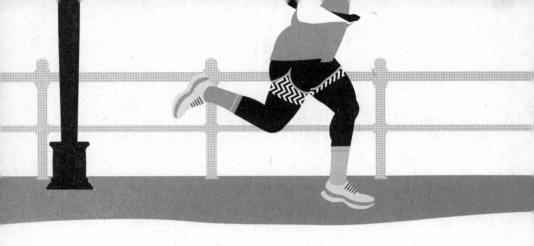

14

Get a gait analysis

Something I'd recommend is a gait analysis. This is one of the first things Babs did for me but it doesn't need to be done by a coach, any number of running shops that sell specialist footwear will do it for you. They are usually staffed by knowledgeable sales professionals who are qualified to advise on the right kind of footwear for your needs.

In running terms, a gait analysis is an assessment of the way the body moves when running; how the foot lands and where. Typically, you do this on a treadmill in the shop, wearing a neutral shoe (a shoe that doesn't offer any special support). It's usually recorded and then played back to you in slow-mo, going frame by frame. The sales rep watches it to help determine whether or not you have any biomechanical misalignments or problems in your ankles or knees.

In my gait analysis, Babs said that I was heavily **over-pronating** and that until I strengthened my arches all the pretty, fashionable running footwear that I had been dabbling with was not for me.

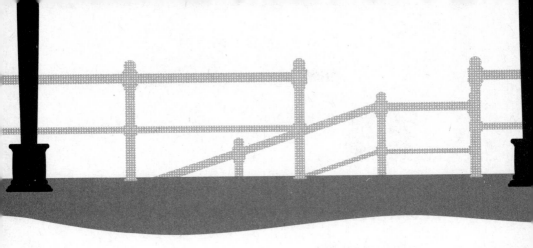

I needed footwear with a little more support, but not too much support as I didn't want to become dependent on it.

Over-pronating is when your foot rolls excessively inwards, transferring all your weight to the inner edge of your foot. It is most often seen in people with low arches or flat feet. I was a big over-pronator because I had very low arches, which is also one of the reasons I would get a certain pain in my feet so frequently (this was plantar fasciitis; I'll tell you more about this common running injury in Chapter 7 on pages 183–5).

Your gait analysis can also reveal whether you **supinate** when you run, which is when the outer side of the foot hits the ground with little or no inward movement. This is normally seen in people with high arches.

Neutral pronation is when the foot lands on the outer edge and rolls inward in a controlled manner. A manner that's just right, a manner that distributes your weight as it should be distributed, helping to absorb all the force from your landing.

Once you've had this done you are in a better place to pick shoes according to your running gait; the sales rep will be able to point you in the right direction. Remember, not all shoes are created equal and not every shoe is right for everyone; they can help or hinder. Your running shoes are important, and making more informed decisions is part of your journey to getting better and better as a runner.

15

Meditation and positive affirmations

I have always likened meditation to tapping into what lies within, a moment where you are consciously flicking a switch in your head, plugging into something deeper. I know this all sounds a bit like Neo in *The Matrix*, but that's what it feels like to me, like I've connected to something different and it's flooding my brain. It's calm.

It often starts with a shallowing of the breath and an acknowledgement that it's time to be in the moment while being elsewhere. This could happen as I'm walking home from work and I know I'll be running soon; it could happen when I'm tying up my laces or when I'm at the start line. It's peaceful. I thank whoever I need to thank for giving me the strength to continue doing what I do and breathe once again. I give myself a little pep talk or repeat a few words, or as some might say a **positive affirmation** – a positive phrase or statement that's used to challenge negative, unhelpful thoughts. It can be as simple as I AM STRONG or I WILL KEEP GOING or I AM IN CONTROL. It's whatever works for you.

My go-to positive affirmation is often FEAR NOT THE WAVE, FOR THE WAVE IS WITHIN YOU, which means the only thing you should be scared of is yourself — and why would you be scared of yourself? If there's nothing or no one to be afraid of but yourself, and you're in control, there's nothing that will stop you from doing what needs to be done but you. So get out of your own way, Cory, get out of your own way. GOT THIS, DONE THIS, GO.

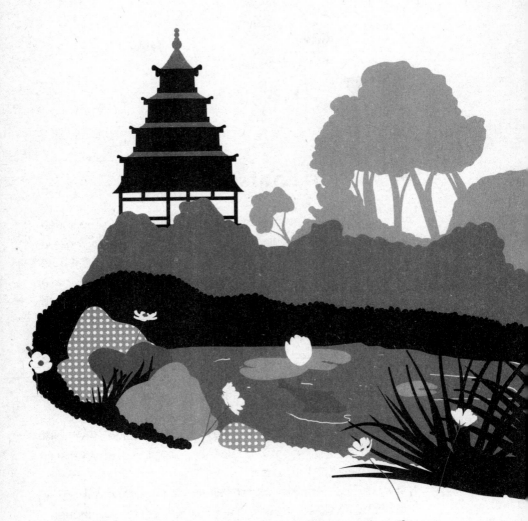

Regardless of how loud everything else is, when I say this affirmation to myself it sounds muffled, like someone had brought the
volume right down: all I can hear is my breath, those words and
my heart. Even in a crowded corral at big race meets I somehow
manage to silence the sounds. The more I ran, the more I realised
that in the end, regardless of how big the team is, it will always be just
you and your breath. Positive affirmations offer me a way to calm
my mind, something that has helped me GET BETTER.

16

Push your limits

A few years back I was running as part of a relay team in The Speed Project; it's an event where you run 340 miles from LA to Vegas in a team of 6 to 12. I honestly didn't do enough training for it but I was fit enough to do it without hurting myself. I had already run a lot that day, not slept much, I was hungry and dehydrated. But that's what I signed up for, so until it was over there was work to be done.

It was the middle of the night and we were coming through what felt like *Breaking Bad* territory, so let's just say the backdrop had an eerie, intimidating feel to it. It didn't help that I had just been woken up to run my leg of the race, so I was really spaced out. It was pitch black, no streetlights, just the light from the team support vehicle behind me. The RV was filled with supplies and other team members, most of whom were sleeping, trying to get their rest in before it was their turn to run.

It was *soooo* hot and humid and all I could think of was taking my top off. I wasn't keen on anyone seeing my stomach, but I thought, hey, it's dark, it will be me and the moon's little secret. I took off my vest and carried it in my hand, sometimes using it to dab the sweat on my chest, doing my best not to get anywhere near my already chafed and bloody nipples and just ran (I know, it sounds bad — see Chapter 7 on injuries). When I write things like this it feels like I'm there. I'm not saying that I'm crying, but boy oh boy do I remember that feeling.

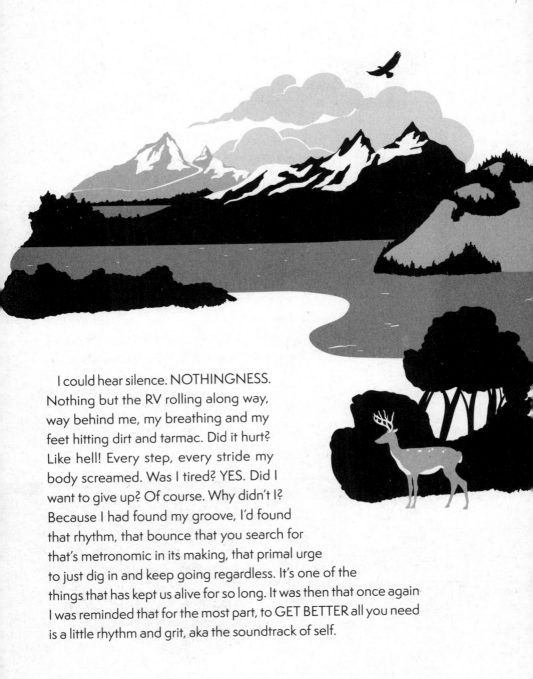

I could hear silence. NOTHINGNESS. Nothing but the RV rolling along way, way behind me, my breathing and my feet hitting dirt and tarmac. Did it hurt? Like hell! Every step, every stride my body screamed. Was I tired? YES. Did I want to give up? Of course. Why didn't I? Because I had found my groove, I'd found that rhythm, that bounce that you search for that's metronomic in its making, that primal urge to just dig in and keep going regardless. It's one of the things that has kept us alive for so long. It was then that once again I was reminded that for the most part, to GET BETTER all you need is a little rhythm and grit, aka the soundtrack of self.

17

Try different types of runs

As a new runner you'll probably have focused on finding a comfortable running pace, and tried to increase it in length and speed gradually when it felt right. But as it turns out, there are many different ways to run. I remember asking lots of questions and concluding that ways of running can be broken down into a few types. All of them can help you become a better runner. Some runs can be combined and some should be done alone. But they all work together. Running is like a puzzle and these are some of the pieces that you can use to form a more detailed picture. It's like when you

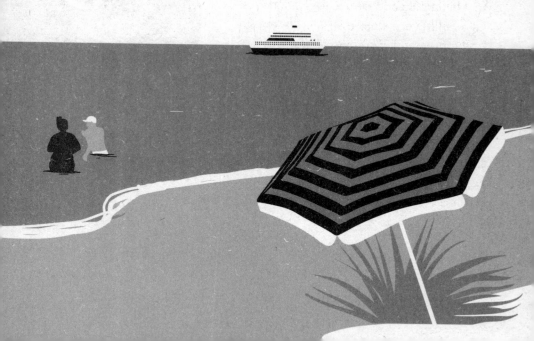

create a player on a video game, each activity you do adds a little star to your overall running ability. Some are better for speed, some for strength, some help with balance and coordination, others with endurance and mental strength. But all help you progress to becoming a more rounded runner.

See Chapter 5 for a detailed rundown of different types of runs. Aim to try some or all of these runs and work them into your run plan. I have my favourites, of course! Try them out and find yours.

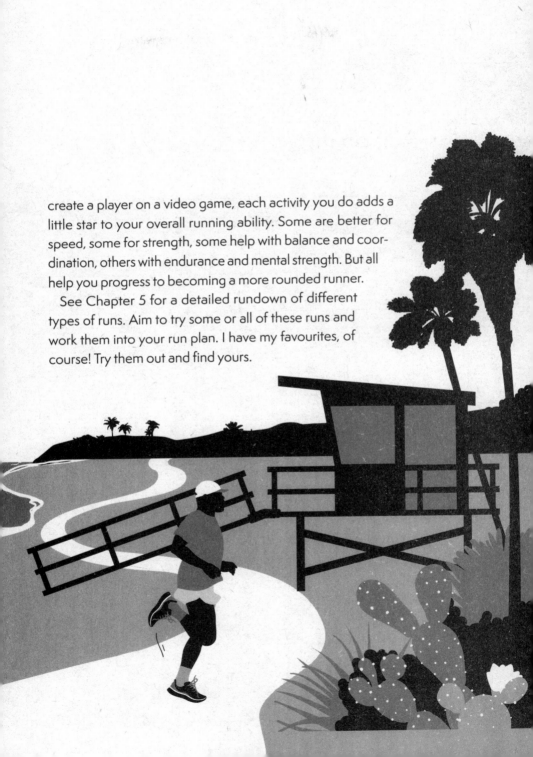

18

Run on different terrains

Strength work in the gym is all well and good, but you can also get stronger – and faster – by running on different terrains, something Coach Babs recommended I do. You can try trail races, trail runs, cross-country runs, road runs, mixed-terrain runs; they all make running more exciting, more engaging, more fun.

Running on different terrains, combining roads and treadmills with trails, is great at challenging you to be a stronger, more aware runner. Roads and treadmills are good at honing your strength,

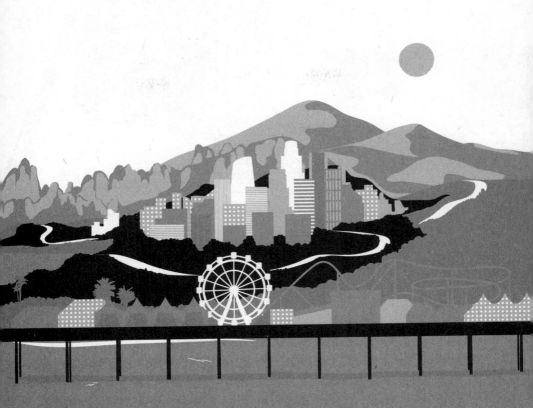

stamina and speed, while trail runs pump up your awareness and agility. You do a lot more work than when you're on the road or treadmill because you have to be ready for incline changes and uneven ground. Running on unexpected, inconsistent surfaces makes your brain work harder to plan your body's reaction, honing your proprioception, your body's ability to sense movement, action and location. (See Chapter 8 for more on Trail Running.) Running on a variety of terrains is key to making you a better runner in every way.

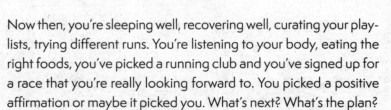

19

Have a plan

Now then, you're sleeping well, recovering well, curating your playlists, trying different runs. You're listening to your body, eating the right foods, you've picked a running club and you've signed up for a race that you're really looking forward to. You picked a positive affirmation or maybe it picked you. What's next? What's the plan?

How many days a week are you going to run? And on what days? What does the mileage look like? At what pace will you be running these miles? Will you be doing speed work? Or track? Running up hills? Down hills? Will you be cross-training? Doing yoga? Pilates? Core? So many things to think about, but don't get overwhelmed: take your time and take one step at a time. I integrated all these things gradually.

A plan helps to give you and your running structure, which helps you organise your life, letting you know in advance what the nutritional needs of your week might be if, for example, you know you've got a long 20-mile run on Sunday. You know you'll be needing a few extra carbs, but you also know that you shouldn't really be out partying all night on Friday or Saturday.

I slowly turned the screw and the first part of it was a basic running plan, one that tells you when to run, how long for in time or distance, and when to rest. In the beginning, that's all you need, and you can keep using it until you want to add more. As time passes and as you see fit, you can work your way up to a plan that incorporates more things from the magic list above. It you want to know what that looks like, I've included some sample plans opposite.

Early Run Plan

WEEK 1

Monday	1 mile
Tuesday	Rest
Wednesday	2 miles
Thursday	Rest
Friday	1 mile
Saturday	Rest
Sunday	3 miles

Weekly Mileage: 7 miles

WEEK 2

Monday	1 mile
Tuesday	Rest
Wednesday	3 miles
Thursday	Rest
Friday	1 mile
Saturday	Rest
Sunday	3 miles

Weekly Mileage: 8 miles

WEEK 3

Monday	2 miles
Tuesday	Rest
Wednesday	2 miles
Thursday	Rest
Friday	2 miles
Saturday	Rest
Sunday	3 miles

Weekly Mileage: 9 miles

WEEK 4

Monday	Rest
Tuesday	Rest
Wednesday	2 miles
Thursday	Rest
Friday	1 mile
Saturday	Rest
Sunday	3 miles

Weekly Mileage: 6 miles

More challenging run plan

In the beginning I got many plans from trawling the internet or in running magazines, running books, YouTube, interviews, running communities, running friends or just by asking people that knew more than me. I wanted to find out what everyone else was doing and how it worked for them.

WEEK 1

Mon	1 mile	EASY
Tue	Active Recovery	Yoga
Wed	2 miles	TEMPO
Thur	Active Recovery	Strength & Core
Fri	1 mile	HILLS
Sat	Rest	
Sun	3 miles	EASY

Weekly Mileage: 7 miles

WEEK 2

Mon	1 mile	EASY
Tue	Active Recovery	Yoga
Wed	3 miles	½ mile EASY, ½ Mile HARD, REPEAT 3X
Thur	Active Recovery	Strength & Core
Fri	1 mile	HILLS
Sat	Rest	
Sun	3 miles	EASY

Weekly Mileage: 8 miles

When I started to incorporate more detail, the same plan might have looked like this instead. The runs are more specific and attention is paid to intensity (see Chapter 5 for more info on the types of runs listed here). On non-run days, rest is mixed with active recovery activities such as yoga and other workouts (see p.126 for strength and core workouts).

WEEK 3

Mon	2 miles	MODERATE
Tue	Active Recovery	Yoga
Wed	2 miles	½ mile EASY, 1 mile HARD, ½ mile EASY
Thur	Active Recovery	Strength & Core
Fri	2 miles	EASY
Sat	Rest	
Sun	3 miles	1½ miles EASY, 1½ miles HARD

Weekly Mileage: 9 miles

WEEK 4

Mon	Rest	
Tue	Active Recovery	Yoga
Wed	2 miles	EASY
Thur	Active Recovery	Strength & Core
Fri	1 mile	MODERATE
Sat	Rest	
Sun	3 miles	EASY

Weekly Mileage: 6 miles

20

Upgrade your running kit

The same thing can be said for the right running kit. Do you know the saying 'There's no such thing as bad weather, only unsuitable clothing'? Well, never was it more true than for your running gear. The more you run, the better you will get at knowing yourself and your body and the kit that you need for certain conditions. In the beginning, when the goal is just to start running by getting yourself out the door, it doesn't really matter. But when you are getting serious, the right clothing can really help you, and it doesn't have to mean dropping your savings into it.

The right kit will help you manage your body temperature – how hot you are, how cold you are, how wet you are, whether it be from rain or sweat. Think about it like this: you wouldn't run through the Sahara Desert where it's 100-plus degrees during the day wearing a Gore-Tex rain jacket, waterproof bottoms and Gore-Tex shoes, would you? For one, you'd be very hot, two, you'd be very sweaty, and three, due to all that sweating you'd be losing a lot of fluid and a lot of salts that would lead to dehydration far more quickly than if you were running in split shorts and vest. The same can be said for the opposite extreme: you wouldn't be wearing split shorts and a vest if you were running through Antarctica in the dead of winter when it's minus 100 degrees as you'd be too cold to move. I have been caught out many times due to poor prep – London winters can be cold! So don't be like me, think about kit early. I'd say there are some essential pieces that every runner should have if they plan to run all year round in varying weather conditions. They don't have to be fancy, but I think having one of each of these will help you be more comfortable when running. And if you are comfortable you might be more likely to create positive memories, which could make you feel like you want to do this running thing a little more.

All of these items should serve a purpose and

>> **Summer and spring:** Short shorts, vest/singlet or short-sleeve tee, short, long or compression socks.

>> **Winter:** Running tights, long-sleeved top, padded vest, rain jacket, gloves, thicker jacket, short, long or compression socks and hat.

FINISH

should either be good at wicking away moisture and keeping you cool or keeping you warm without overheating. You'll find that many sportswear outlets and high-street shops have their own-brand sportswear section that you can get items from if you don't want to spend *tooooo* much money. Also think about intelligently layering when you're out on a run, allowing you to add or take off clothes depending on how you're feeling and on the ever-changing weather conditions. This is especially important when you start heading out for longer runs.

You might also want to think about getting a running bag that straps around your stomach. It's basically a bum bag made for running or, as

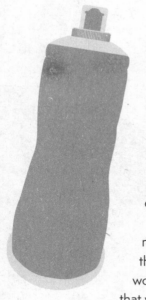

the Americans call it, a fanny pack. You can put your keys, cards, gels, etc. in it, meaning your hands will be free to propel you on to greatness. Of course, you could put all of these things in your pockets, depending on how much you're carrying. If it's just keys and card they can go in the back or side pocket, but anything heavier tends to be a little off-putting and can mess with the rhythm of your arm drive and stride over longer periods of time.

The longer and further you run the more gels you will need, and there will come a point and time where the all the gels just won't fit into the little bag. At that point you would go for a running belt. This has ten or so little holes that you can slot your gels into. The hardest part is getting them in without them popping. If you're really fancy, get one that has the bum-bag part and lots of holes for gels.

You can also get an armband phone holder that wraps around your bicep.

If you don't fancy any of that, you can get yourself a good old-fashioned running backpack that you can load up with whatever it is that you need to carry.

When it comes to carrying water you have a number of options. A camel pack is a backpack with a bag in it that you fill with water or any other drink. The long flexible tube loops out the backpack and is easily accessible for when you want a sip. Or you can go for bottles that slip into a running belt, or hand-held bottles you can put your hands through and grip easily.

I have at one point or another in my running life used all of the things that I have mentioned and the only one I don't really use or get on with is the armband. Everything else I loved. Remember, it's a personal choice, so find what works for you.

Once, in the midst of my own marathon training, I was running with a group of friends that I regularly coached but also trained with. On this occasion it was a jump in, jump out run, meaning it was one long route of around 20 miles and people jumped in and out depending on what mileage they were looking for. Some people would start out with me and jump out at mile 5 or 10, others might jump in at mile 5 or 10 and jump out at 15 or stay with me to the end. This run was ridiculous as I was out running for four hours plus. I kicked off at Shoreditch station, hit the canals till we reached the Thames, ran through the city, through central London and back east, and the weather just kept changing. Rain, cold, sleet, sun, warm, back to cold, nope, warm

I was able to warm up when I needed to and let my body breathe when I needed to.

again. It was four seasons in a day. What saved me? INTELLIGENT LAYERING. I was able to warm up when I needed to and let my body breathe when I needed to. So all I had to worry about was making sure I had enough energy to keep going. Which actually leads nicely into learning how to FUEL ON THE GO.

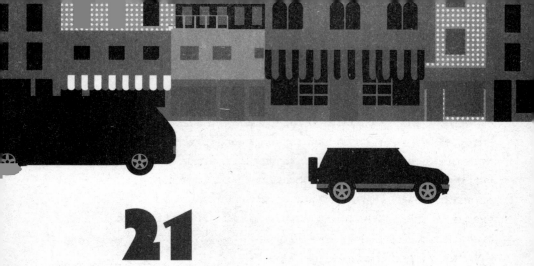

21

Learn to fuel on the go

Now when I say FUEL ON THE GO I mean eating or drinking something mid-run to give you the energy to keep going when you start to get tired. This could be a gel, sweets, fruits or some other snack – all those simple carbs I mentioned earlier. Come race day, or when you're training for a race, you need to be able to get that energy on board quickly so you don't stop completely at each station, breaking your flow. You never see marathon runners stopping for a cup of tea and a biscuit, do you?

If I'm running for 90 minutes or less I just run on what's in my stomach.

Now, I love using gels but it helps to practise with them, or whatever fuel you are using, during training; don't wait until race day. Use some trial and error to figure out what works for you. I have personally tried ten to twenty different types of gels, sports drinks and other foods, like rice balls, cold pasta, chocolate bars, sweets, potatoes and fruit. The list is endless . . . All in a bid to find out what works for me and to find out how often I need to take them.

In the beginning I was surprised at how many gels gave me

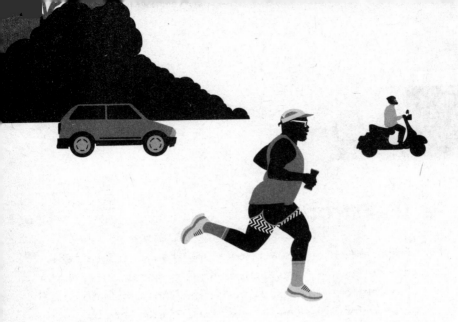

stomach cramps and gastric distress – my body told me pretty quickly to get to a toilet immediately lol. This is quite common if you don't find the gel that's right for you. Sadly, these consequences are *ooooooooh*, too familiar to me. One year it happened when I was running the London Marathon. I either had a dodgy gel or just too many of them and my body said *evacuate, evacuate*. And that was more or less the end of my race with 17 miles to go. I still finished, just a little less energetically than I'd hoped . . .

As the years have passed, I have found a handful of specific gels that work for me. Most races offer water and some kind of electrolytes like Lucozade or Gatorade as well as fruit, but I know they probably won't be handing out the gels on the course that work for me, so I run with my gels either in a little bum bag or a gel belt where I can store five to ten of them. If I'm running for 90 minutes or less I just run on what's in my stomach; for anything after that I'll plan fuelling accordingly. Do your research and decide what works for you. I've seen people dip pizza in Coca Cola . . . It's not something I've tried personally, but, like I say, everyone's different.

22

Get stronger

Using gels and other snacks to fuel you when you're tired is effective, but improving your running efficiency means you can run for longer before getting tired – this is something Coach Babs worked on with me. You achieve better running efficiency by getting stronger and working on your mobility, flexibility and balance. *All* can not only improve your efficiency but also work towards preventing injuries.

Now, when I say getting stronger, I mean getting stronger *everywhere*, not just in your legs but your whole body. While you're trying to get stronger, think about body weight and resistance exercises as well as strength. Don't try and turn your workout into a CrossFit or hybrid cardio workout, as I'm sure you get more than enough of that from your running and any other cross-training activities you might be doing.

Babs had me doing body weight exercises aswell as exercises with weights and other equipment. These movements would involve multiple joints and muscle groups, all of which are used when running. Doing these exercises helped me become a stronger, faster, more efficient runner — THAT'S THE GOAL.

Try the following exercises — you can make them more challenging by adding weight, spending more time under tension or by adding small movements and little pulses. Try building some or all of these into your weekly routine.

Lunges

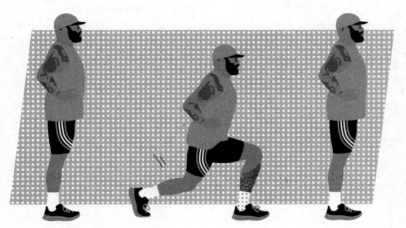

Lunges strengthen the glutes (aka your bum muscle), your hamstrings which run down the back of your legs, your quads which are the set of big muscle groups on the front of your upper leg, and your calves which are the muscles at the back and top of your lower leg, beneath your knee pit. You get a lot of bang for your buck with lunges as they also work your core and lower back, which help to keep you stable as you lunge and when you are stationary.

The beauty of the lunge is there are so many variations that can make it easier or harder, or just different. Lunges to the front, the back, the side. Lunges with weights by your side, over your head, out wide. Supported lunges, lunges onto an unstable or uneven surface like a bosu ball (a balance platform that looks like a big exercise ball cut in half with a flat underside) or wobble board — *sooooo* many options and each works the body in a slightly different way. But all help to improve your range of motion, especially in the hip area where runners tend to be tight – me especially.

Start off with a **standard lunge** to make sure you get the form right and then move into **walking lunges**, which are dynamic and act as an exaggerated form of running. They also require balance and coordination which is key to running too, when you're either pushing off one foot and landing on the other or both feet are in the air floating along. The only time both feet are on the floor is when you are still, so it would make sense to replicate that movement where you can.

Make sure you have the form right: feet hip-width apart, core engaged, chest up. Step forward with your left leg, keeping your right leg where it is. Bend both your knees so your legs are at a 90-degree angle. Make sure your left knee (lead leg) does not push forward past your toes, and your right knee (back leg) is hovering above the ground. From the side it should look like your shin and back are making the same lines. Hold for a few seconds. Brace, push through your front heel, come back to standing and repeat on the other leg.

In the beginning I did sets of anywhere from 5 to 20 lunges on each leg and anywhere between 2 and 4 sets.

For **lateral lunges**, look straight ahead, stand tall, feet together, chest up, shoulders back. Take a big step to your left, hinge forward at the hips, sit back a little as if trying to sit on a chair. Bend your left knee into a lunge position. Hold or pulse. Push off your left foot and return to the start position. Switch legs. REPEAT.

By doing lateral lunges you also target the adductors. These are the muscles on your inner thighs that you use to close your legs. (I used to pay special attention to my adductors because before meeting Coach Babs every marathon I ever ran I cramped up right there and it was *absolute agony*.)

My favourite lunge variation is the walking lunge holding two kettle bells by my side, one in each arm. I used to do walking lunges up and down Babs's studio till she said STOP. At times I was sure her stopwatch had broken because though she said a minute it felt like five.

Your legs might tingle and burn after only a few lunges, but as time passes you'll grow in strength and be able to do more. It's one of the things that I really liked about working with Babs. I could literally see and feel myself improving. And with that improvement I prayed for no more cramp – and thankfully, my prayers were answered.

Squats

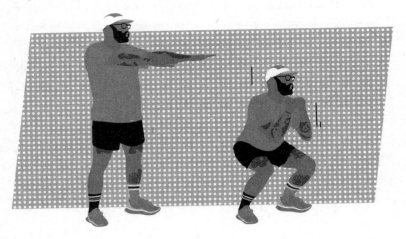

Next up we hit the squats, aka the movement we go through to sit down and stand up. The squat is really effective as it works the glutes, hamstrings, quads, calves, core *and* adductors and can be done with just your body weight. Or you can be assisted, e.g. by holding onto something, or you can add weights.

Before you do these, double check you're sitting and standing correctly to prevent injury. As ever, get the form right. Keep your head and chest up looking straight ahead. Shoulders relaxed, core engaged, making sure to keep a neutral spine, meaning don't lean forwards or back and don't round your spine. Now try sitting on the edge of a chair, box or bench, one that is just below your knees. Put your hands on your hips, make sure your feet are shoulder width apart, pointing forwards. Or if you need to work on your mobility like me, you can take a wider stance.

Squeeze your bum to engage your glutes and push up till you are standing. Sit down nice and slowly, making sure your knees don't buckle inwards on the way down, and repeat. Once you think you've got your form locked, try doing it without the bench, box or chair.

You know you've got the perfect squat form when your nose, knees and toes are all pointing in the same direction. I do anywhere between one and three sets of 10–15 reps with recovery in between.

I have to say my favourite squat variation is a squat with a kettle bell in one hand that I hold by my head. After coming up from the squat I press that one arm over my head. I do that five times before switching to the other side, then take a rest and repeat.

Step-ups

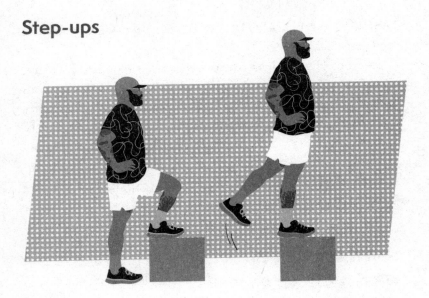

Next, step-ups – and I know some of you might be reading this and thinking *huhhhhhh*, step-ups, how is this here with squats and lunges? Well, I'm here to tell you step-ups are very underrated.

I remember doing step-ups onto a box facing a wall for 45 minutes straight . . . It should have been 60 minutes but I was told they needed the wall 😊. This was all in a bid to help strengthen my legs as I was on my way back from an injury and couldn't yet run. But I had a race coming up that I could still be ready for if I concentrated on maintaining cardio and strength. Step-ups were a valuable piece of the puzzle. You'll be happy to know that I didn't just reserve step-ups for the facing walls, I did them everywhere. Don't be like me — DON'T DO STEP-UPS FOR 45 MINUTES FACING A WALL, IT'S LUDICROUS lol. But the things we do are the things we do.

A sensible amount of step-ups to start off with would be more like 2–4 sets of 6–10 step-ups on each leg. You can either do them with just your body weight, or you can add weight. And if you want a little extra bang for your buck you can add a knee drive at the top of the movement. Just BE CAREFUL. Only do that if you feel comfortable and you are BALANCED.

Step-ups of any variation help to increase strength in your legs, even out imbalances, strengthen your core and improve your balance. And you guessed it, these li'l step-ups work your quads, hammies, calves, glutes and adductors.

Be careful. Only do that if you feel comfortable and you are balanced.

The way to do a step-up properly is to find a step or box that you are comfortable stepping up and down from. It could be as low as shoe box or as high as your hips. Stand *tall* in front of said step or box. Keep your head up, chest up, shoulders back, looking straight ahead. Place your right foot on your step or box making sure on that side your hip, knee and ankle are all at 90 degrees. Push your body up with your right leg until it's straight. Keep your other leg floating in the air. Take a few seconds then lower back down and switch legs.

When you do this, make sure that the leg that you're stepping with is doing the work and you're not using your other leg for momentum. As you lower your leg, make sure it's nice and controlled.

Hip hinge

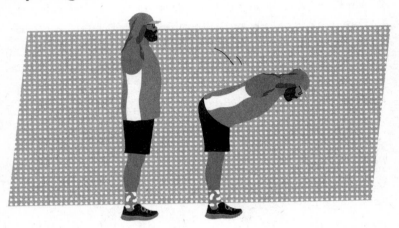

When I first started doing these, Babs would have me stand about a foot from a wall, facing away from it. I'd engage my core, tuck my chin, hinge from my hips, keeping my back straight while pushing my bum backwards till it tapped the wall. This movement helped me learn how to drive my hips back and forth without my spine or knees moving. As time passed and my range of motion improved, I'd inch forward.

When I had the form right, we double checked it by introducing a broomstick, which also helped to really drive home the form. I'd hold the broomstick behind my back making sure it was touching the back of my head, the top of my back and the bottom of my spine near my bum, and then repeat the same hinge movement while the broom maintained contact with those three points: head, upper back and lower back.

After she knew I had it dialled in, weights were introduced – *very, very* LIGHT WEIGHTS. Nothing crazy, no lifting cars or houses, just little kettle bells, as that's all I needed at the time.

I'd place the kettle bell between my legs, feet shoulder width apart. Then hinge just like I had practised with my knees slightly bent. Grab the kettle bell with both hands keeping my arms extended. I'd breathe out quickly and with some gusto while driving my hips forwards, I'd straighten my knees and lift the li'l kettle bell off the floor. To put it down I'd do the same thing in reverse, always making sure my back was straight. I started off with 2–3 sets of 8–12 reps and as time passed I moved onto heavier kettle bells, single-leg kettle bell deadlifts, and a while later a barbell.

Deadlifts

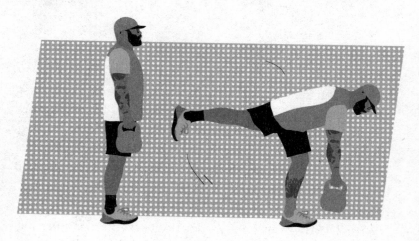

Before attempting these, be sure you master the hip hinge (opposite). Now for deadlifts, which in layman's terms is simply the act of picking up a dead weight from the floor – it's one of the best strength exercises that any runner can do. I say this as we runners tend to suffer from weak glutes, hammies and hips. The deadlift helps to strengthen all of those as well as the core, lower back and much more along the posterior chain, which is a fancy way of saying the backside of your body as opposed to your front side. Strengthening all these muscles can help to reduce lower back pain, improve your posture, and help you run longer and harder with less effort. I mean, come on, who doesn't want that?

As with all of these exercises there are a number of variations. My favourite is definitely the **single-leg kettle bell deadlift**. Like all of these exercises it should be done with good form or you risk injury, especially in situations where you're trying to throw heavy weights around. This is one exercise I really suggest DOING WITH A COACH, or someone who knows what they're doing and better yet what you should be doing.

The single-leg deadlift is great for runners and is a little different to a normal deadlift. You're only on one leg, doing your utmost to turn your body into a T shape, therefore balance comes into things. (Instead of going straight in with weights, I started practising the movement first without any weight.)

Place the kettle bell on the floor in front of you so that you have something to aim for. Then, while keeping a very flat back, put all your weight on your left leg and start to hinge forwards from your hips while bringing your right leg up behind you and trying to touch the kettle bell with your right hand, all at the same time. As I said, this is a great exercise for balance and coordination. Do 5 on each side, rest and repeat 3 times.

Strengthening all these muscles can help to reduce lower back pain, improve your posture, and help you run longer and harder.

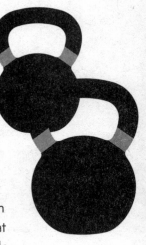

Box jumps

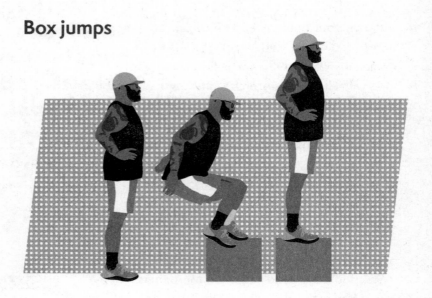

Another favourite exercise of mine is box jumps, which actually helped me generate a li'l extra torque or power in my running stride, the reason being box jumps help build your legs and core.

A box jump is exactly what it sounds like, you jump onto a box. The height varies from a shoe box size all the way to silly stuff. I don't know how, but I've seen people jump onto fridges — *you don't need to do that* lol . . . but give them a try. Start small, either in your house on steps or outside on the kerb, or a very small wall, just 3–5 reps, 2–3 sets, and build from there, as too much too soon will blow your calves — and yes, Uncle Cory has blown his calves out from box jumps as I underestimated how much plyometric exercises like that (see pages 197–8) work the body. *But*, as with all things, when not overdone they help to make you stronger.

Med ball slams and balance work

I love me some med ball slams and balance work on wobble boards or bosu balls. All that balancing helps with the proprioception. A great way to think about proprioception is to imagine turning all the lights off in your house and trying to walk around barefoot. You can't see anything so your feet automatically react to the surroundings; if you step on a shoe or a toy, your feet just know what to do. I started off with balancing on each leg for a few seconds at a time and worked my way up to a minute. At first it was just about standing there and finding my balance. Then as time passed it was about movement, catching, throwing, slamming. Give it a try and don't be afraid to play and experiment.

Med balls (or medicine or exercise balls) are weighted balls about a shoulder width in diameter, and a med ball slam is when you pick one up and slam it on the floor. The child in me loves throwing stuff, so I really enjoy this exercise. It's tiring because it works your whole body, especially your hips, core, shoulders and back, which are areas that we forget are also important. We talk a lot about strengthening the lower body, but the upper body is just as important because that's where your arm drive comes from. And, believe it or not, your arm drive can act as another set of legs helping to drive you onwards.

Upper body exercises

As I've just suggested, please don't neglect the upper body! With weights I do single-arm bent-over rows with light dumbbells as well as overhead presses. The press uses your lower back, upper back, arms and shoulders, and the row works all those muscles as well as your hips, side body, biceps and triceps, which are key to running. The single-arm bent-over row movement always reminds me of how I would use a really heavy handsaw to cut wood.

I originally did all of these exercises under the supervision of people who knew more than me or by watching those who knew more than me. Practice can make perfect but only if you're practicing the right thing. So if you do try any of them I suggest you do the same, either with a coach, a trainer in the gym, or an app like Apple Fitness+ that can help you mix up your running with cross-training. And depending on which workout you pick you might even see me getting my cross-train on .

All of these exercises really helped me get better as a runner. I literally felt stronger, my core felt tighter, I felt more supported in the later miles in races, I could maintain better form and wouldn't get fatigued as quickly. I felt a little bit like a puppet whose strings had been pulled a little tighter, and after a while when I walked I was floating, not because I was *godly* or a *spirit* but because I was STRONG.

There are so many other exercises and so many variations that I could talk about, but the ones I've mentioned here are those I really worked on and paid me back. I hope they'll do wonders for you, too.

23

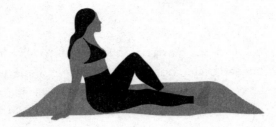

Try movement classes

You're probably thinking to yourself, hold on, I thought running was just about running. And it can be, but if it is you miss out on so much more. As if all the above wasn't enough, one of the other things that I think is a must is **yoga**. It has helped me with my overall strength, my core, range of motion and flexibility. It has not only helped to strengthen my big muscles but also the tiny li'l underused muscles, tendons and ligaments that help to support them. That also helps to reduce the possibility of injuries.

Range of motion is important, as it can help save energy. I'm going to use fake numbers here just to prove a point: imagine every stride I take covers only 1 metre, but every stride you take covers 2 metres. That means that you are hitting the ground half as many times as me to cover the same distance, using half as much energy.

When it comes to improving your flexibility, think about it this way: that improvement can decrease the likelihood of injury due to strains and tears in your muscles and ligaments. Something that I can 100 per cent attest to as I noticed, when I'm deep into yoga, doing it three or four times a week, I feel STRONG and FLEXIBLE. Yoga also helps with my breathing, so why not give it a try and don't be shy. And if yoga isn't for you, there are alternatives like Pilates, which is often referred to as 'yoga's more athletic cousin', and Barre, a workout that incorporates ballet-inspired movements focused on challenging your balance and building strength. All can help with your breathing.

I know all of these things can be intimidating, and the first step is the hardest. So why not share that step with a friend and get stronger and better together? And if, for example, you don't want to go to a class with a friend, or they're not available, let the studio know you're a newbie, let them know you may need help. It's something that I have done at every studio I have gone to, as I know my body doesn't do what I want it to.

've shared a range of ideas for stepping it up once you're past the uber-beginner-runner stage. These are the steps I took and the things I tried, and I hope you'll try some or all of them, too.

A final word on self-care – maybe you don't need telling, but the importance of investing in self-care is underrated. Running, and training your body to be a better runner, brings its rewards but it can be hard work at times. So look after yourself – book a massage, do a steam, do a sauna, try acupuncture if you want to. Acupuncture points are believed to stimulate the central nervous system and this stimulation helps to release chemicals into the body and brain, which may help to stimulate the body's natural healing abilities. In my years of running I have had acupuncture many times and I must say, it works for me. I won't deny it's an added cost, but when you're putting your body through the mill, all of these things help to keep the body ticking over.

Since I started taking running seriously, since it has become more than my passion but also my job, I have a minimum of one massage a week. It helps to release tension in my muscles, improves my range of motion and helps to speed up the recovery and healing process of banged-up muscles. You don't have to do it weekly, but try it once and see if it helps. A sports massage will target specific areas and a

Swedish massage can help you relax. If you really want to get into the knots, try a Thai massage.

And if you want to add a little cherry on top of all this, something that will really help you become a better runner is simple:

BE A SPONGE.

Immerse yourself in running culture, whatever part of it you choose, it's up to you. You can go to running club meets and races, bigger more mainstream races like the London Marathon. You can go and watch cross-country, track races, road running, go to seminars, retreats out in the trails, you can run relays. The lifestyle and culture of running is anything and everything that is associated with this sport I love. It might even be things that we don't think about, like where do runners eat? What coffee do they drink and why? There's a whole world out there, and now you've started to run you can jump in and explore.

Maybe you don't need telling, but the importance of investing in self-care is underrated.

A lot of the things that I know to be true, things that have helped me, I have picked up from either asking questions, seeing things happen or just by being in the room. So read, read, read, look and listen, as there's a lot of free information being handed out based on real-life experience. Some of it should be taken with a grain of salt, and I'm sure you know not everyone's body is the same. But find or build a community and IMMERSE yourself in the running world. You won't regret it.

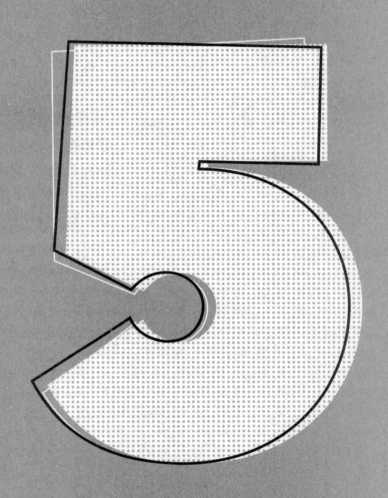

The Rundown

Different types of runs

n the beginning, I'd just run to the end of the road and back. Then I started running around the block and, when I was ready, I ran longer routes around town, before my little legs took me all over the world. But the thing is, regardless of where I was on this magical journey, I was always just running, trying to find a rhythm and getting into the swing of moving my arms and legs, breathing enough to run without passing out, and aiming to reach a point where it hurt less and less until it felt good. And when it felt good, I pushed a little harder till it hurt all over again.

That's the beauty of running: you can push, or you can hold. It's always your call. In the previous chapter one of my suggestions for helping you become a better runner is to try different types of runs. Did you know there are many ways to run? I'll tell you about them here.

Base pace

When I first started, and when many others start, all you do is run base pace runs as it's the only pace you really know – whether it's once a week or three or four times a week.

This run is your base, a pace that your body naturally slips into without trying, a pace that's conversational. No heavy breathing or panicking – it should literally feel like a walk in the park. As time passes a short run like this should feel somewhat effortless. If it doesn't, then you're trying too hard and going too fast . . . Slow down.

Even Olympians and world champions spend the bulk of their time running at their base pace. It's at this pace that you build endurance and strength in your legs as your body gets used to being on its feet. It's at this base pace that you work on your running efficiency, which is how much energy you burn with each step you take. The better your running efficiency, the less energy you burn as you move and the more energy you have for going faster or longer when the time is right. The beauty of the base pace run is it's ever-changing. The fitter you get, the stronger you get, the quicker your base pace will become. If you've had a rough night or haven't got as much sleep as usual or your nutrition is off, your base pace will be a little slower.

Progressive build

Next up, progressive build runs or, simply, progression runs. This is the type of run where you start off at your natural pace and progressively get faster over the course of the run, or just finish faster than you started. This run is a little bit harder than your base pace. It's a great way to introduce getting faster without doing a tempo or interval run, which we will talk about shortly.

When I started I would set out at my normal base pace, say for a 30-minute run. Give it a try. At the 10-minute mark, when you've started to feel a little warmer, up the pace a little bit – and I really mean a little bit. When I first started doing these I would run at a 10-minute mile pace and when I first picked up my pace would only increase to 9:50 or 9:45 per mile. When you hit the 20-minute mark, pick it up again if you can. Once again, when I picked it up my pace would increase from 9:50 to 9:45 or from 9:45 to 9:30. You can pick a number, whichever number you like as long as it's a li'l quicker. The purpose is to get your body used to running a little bit quicker for longer periods of time without adding too much speed. You'll find that by doing this more often, your base pace will get quicker.

Fartlek runs

Once you've got used to running a little bit quicker on your runs, a great way to continue improving is to progress and try out fartlek runs. Fartlek is Swedish for speed play, so you'll do just that: play with speed. It's a type of interval that has no set time or distance. A great way to start working on being even more efficient when you run. It starts to get you and your body used to managing a little bit of discomfort at quicker speeds.

Fartlek is great for everyone but especially for beginners; unlike tempo runs or traditional intervals you get to do what you like. You get to pick up the pace when you want and slow down when you want. This is probably the type of run that I have had the most fun with, as there are no rules. I would take groups out on runs and simply say, 'Okay, see that bench in the distance? We are going to run hard to it when the light turns green.' Or, 'Let's pick up the pace to make the light.' Or we'd pick up the pace when we saw a green car and slow it down when we saw a red car. You're not sprinting, just upping the pace a little.

Another great way to do fartleks is to use music: run easy on the verses and hard on the chorus. Or run easy on the main roads and hard on the backstreets. These types of runs build speed, and stamina as well, as they keep you fresh and can be done for any amount of time. Your rules.

My favourite place to play fartlek was a long road that led from London's Marble Arch, down Bayswater Road, onto Holland Park and finally into Shepherd's Bush. This straight road was littered with traffic lights. My game was simple: You have to get from one end to the other. If you see a green light you keep running, if it's red you turn round and go back to the light before. So instead of you choosing what pace to run at, the lights are in charge of what you do. You pick up the pace if you see a light might be changing. I have

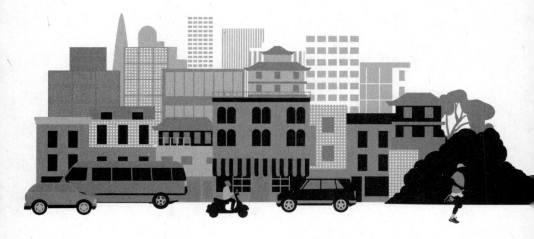

seen people get all the way to the bottom, they are on the last light and they mistime their sprint and end up having to go way back. It reminds me of snakes and ladders.

Interval runs

Once I'd had some fun with fartlek runs I progressed onto more traditional interval runs or speed workouts, which are another way to build speed and stamina as well as physical and mental strength. An interval run is a run that consists of short bursts of effort, divided out over the course of your run. The interval lasts for a set period of time, it could be anywhere from 15 seconds to 5 minutes and beyond, and it's then followed up with rest for a similar period of time. This can be done anywhere: on the track, on the road, in parks, on trails, etc. One of my favourite interval workouts when I first started is a simple one. I'd warm up for 10–15 minutes at easy pace. I'd then run hard for 30 seconds and easy for 30 seconds. When I started I could only do it for 5 minutes and I'd be dead. After six to eight weeks or so of doing that once a week, I'd worked my way up to be able to do it for 15 minutes and I'd found that my base pace was a little bit quicker.

Track workouts

Running on the track isn't strictly a type of run because you can do a number of different runs on a track – interval runs, for example, are excellent at the track. I am including track runs here because they provide a controlled environment for all kinds of running; the distance doesn't change and if for whatever reason you need to stop you can just step off the track. As I always say to people, why fear the track? You are only ever 400m from SAFETY. I know people are often intimidated by the track, but I honestly think if you follow the rules it's the best place to really hone your running.

Now, you are probably wondering where to find a running track near you if you haven't seen one. Fear not, my friend, they are but a Google away. More often than not they are attached to another facility or club, either a leisure centre, college, school or university. Some are private and you have to be a member. Some are public but you have to be a member of the club to access discounted rates, and others are completely free to use and publicly open to every-one, but they open and close at certain times – so sadly no midnight sessions. The price varies from a few pounds to a few more pounds.

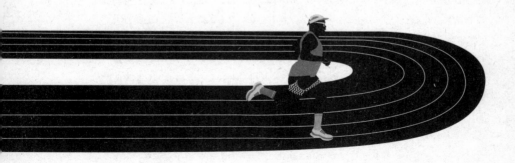

So have a look and see what you find. You might be surprised to find out that after all these years of turning right, if only you'd turned left you would have discovered a track.

When we started our London running group, TrackMafia, it was with the goal of becoming stronger, more efficient runners, so we worked on doing just that. We'd meet once a week, trackside, at 6.30 p.m. on Thursday night and three of us would take the session, taking turns delivering different parts of it. In the beginning the people that came were people who we already knew, people who were part of our little running ecosystem. People who came to the Monday session of the group I'd been running called RDCWest, people who came on long runs, people from work. It sounds like there were lots of people, but in the beginning it was small.

I honestly think if you follow the rules it's the best place to really hone your running.

My friends Jules (later my girlfriend and then my wife) and Jeggi and I started with a simple session at Paddington Recreation Ground that involved 400m reps. Jeggi was the fastest, Jules just behind him, with me bringing up the rear, holding onto Jules and doing my utmost to not get dropped.

You can create your own challenges on the track, incorporating some of the run types I've already listed here, or simply try to improve your lap times. If you'd like something that pushes you to improve strength and speed, the following section offers a track workout similar to what we delivered at TrackMafia. If you find a track you like and can access easily, I really recommend you try this once a week. Recruit a friend or two to do it with you if you want, it'll be more fun.

1

Warm up properly

Start with a 4 lap or 1 mile warm-up at an easy pace, getting your joints, ligaments and muscles well lubricated and working efficiently with one another. Then do another mile or 4 laps but try strides down the straights and jog the bends.

Strides are little bursts of speed or faster running that last 10–20 seconds or 50 metres plus. The idea is to help warm up the body by replicating the thing that you plan to do later in the session, so your body is ready for it. It knows.

Now, this isn't the sort of warm-up I do every time I go for a run – don't get me wrong, if I had all the time in the world I would, but these drills are done specifically to prep the body for running *hard*. You'll find that most of these drills and much of the warm-up is done by professional athletes before they run for their countries and clubs and, of course, break records.

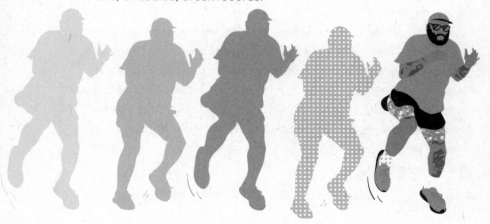

2

Activation drills

After the strides as part of a dynamic warm-up are activation drills. These are a set of low-intensity exercises designed specifically to prepare your body for the more intense activity that will come. Many of these drills replicate what your body will do later on in the workout. This activity also reinforces the connection between your brain and your body. It's like boosting a WiFi or phone signal before making a call or surfing the net.

These drills also help to strengthen your body and get the main muscle groups you'll be using fired up and ready to go to work for you. I would think about getting my brain fired up, as well as the glutes, quads, hamstrings and calves. My routine changed from time to time but these were my go-to drills. I used them for myself as well as when working with or training others. You can find many other coaches and athletes using them in some variation. I find it even more fun when I do these drills to music, doing my utmost to stay on beat while working on my running ABCs – Agility, Balance and Coordination. It makes me feel like I'm in an eighties aerobics video or vibesin' with Mr Motivator. I would do 5–10 of each drill, or do them for anywhere between 15 and 30 seconds each, and I actually created a class called 'Forge' at a gym I used to work at called Ministry Does Fitness that was based solely around these drills and a few others. We would do the class in a little room that reminded me of being at a drum and bass rave, all the flashing lights, disco balls and banging beats.

A

CRUSH GRAPES/FAST FEET

Stand with your feet hip width apart, lower your body ever so slightly into a half squat, and bring your hands out in front of you. Lift your heels up so you're on the balls of your feet, and pretend you're trying to crush grapes beneath your feet. Start off slowly and build in momentum.

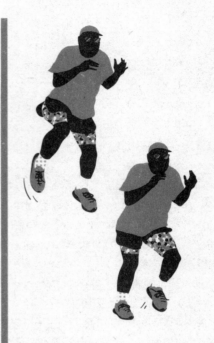

B

LATERAL HOPS

Keep your legs together and jump from side to side as if you're jumping over a shoe box or small hurdle, landing with soft knees and doing your best to land on the balls of your feet. For single-leg lateral hops, do the same but on one leg before switching to the other leg.

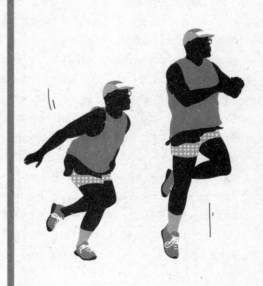

C

LUNGE AND REACH/
LUNGE AND TWIST

Lunge forward. Take a step, not too big or wide, lower your body into a lunge. Reach your right arm up, take a step, switch arms, take a step and raise both arms. Now do the same but instead of reaching up, spread your arms wide and rotate your trunk, doing your best not to over-rotate.

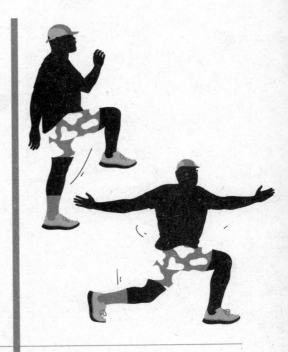

D

CLIFFORD THE CRAB

This is exactly what it sounds like. Make like a crab and scuttle or shuffle, being careful not to roll your ankle. Make sure you change direction and you're not just scuttling in one direction.

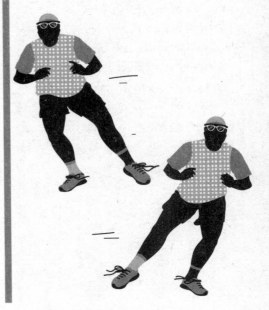

E

GLUTE-PULL WALK

Walk, and with every stride bring one of your legs up. Hold your ankle and knee and pull your ankle and knee towards your chest. Take a step and switch legs.

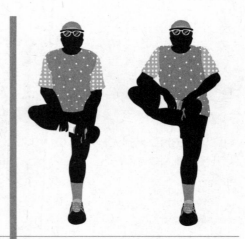

F

MARCH AND GRAB

Take a step and balance on one leg while lifting your other leg, driving upwards with your knee, trying to get it in line with your hips or higher. Engage your core, squeeze the glute of your standing leg, lean forwards towards your standing leg and try to grab something on the floor. Take a step, do the same thing again.

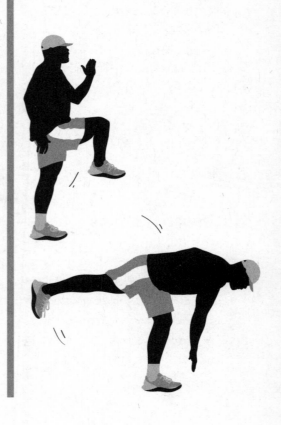

G

GRAPEVINES

Take side steps, and with each step switch between your feet crossing in front of and behind each other.

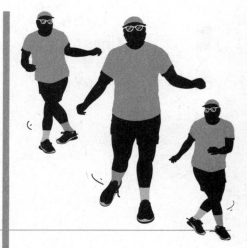

H

LEG SWINGS: LOW, MEDIUM AND HIGH

Look straight ahead. Starting off low (shin height), keep your leg as straight as you can and swing it forward, bounce, then switch legs. Do this a few times before switching to medium (knee to hip height), then to high (hip to head height). Finally, on every swing of your leg get the upper body involved by reaching towards your toe with the opposite arm. If you don't want to bounce, just walk and switch legs every few steps.

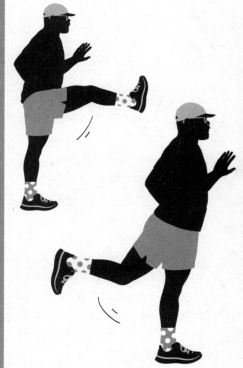

I

HEEL FLICKS

Try and hit your bum with your heel as you walk and then jog.

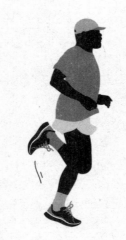

J

HIGH KNEES – A-SKIPS – BEEF KICK – POWER SKIP

Drive your knee up, take a step, switch legs and repeat. After a few of those, add a little bounce or hop as your knee rises, then land on your other foot. After repeating a few more times, if you'd like to make it even more exciting do the same thing but this time as you bring up each leg, raise your arm on the same side as if you were volunteering for something or wanting to answer a question. Now do it all again, but aim for height and not distance.

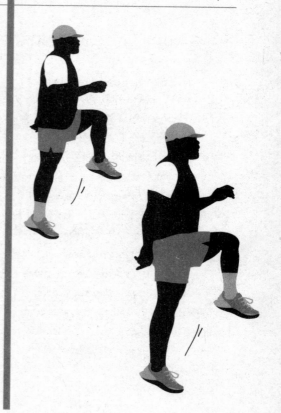

3

The track run

After the warm-up and drills you get into the main
bulk of the session, using the track to hit a specific goal.
Start simple. This goal is individual to you.

For the sake of simple maths let's say *my* goal is to run
a sub 20-minute 5k in a road race that's coming up soon –
that means I would need to run each kilometre at 4 minutes
or below, or 6 minutes 25 seconds for a mile. Or if I break that
down into 400m reps it means I have to be able to run 12½ × 400m
back to back with no break, each in 96 seconds or less. I know that's
a lot of maths and I'm sorry, but that's it for now. If you don't want
to do the maths you can download a pace calculator or use one
online, which is way easier.

So that's my goal. I try to run 4 × 400m on the track at my goal
pace, which is 96 seconds for every 400m lap. I run 4 × 400m then
rest and do another 4 × 400m, on repeat, timing myself each time.
(I picked 4 × 400m as the total distance is 1.6k, which is a pinch under
a mile, so great for pacing.)

To start with, I allow a 60-second recovery in between each
400m rep I do. As the weeks pass I bring the recovery time down
between each 400m rep to 45 seconds, then 30 seconds, then 15
seconds. Then I try and do 2 × 800m at the same pace, starting off
with a 60-second recovery. It's the same 1 mile, but now rather than
being broken in four with four recoveries in between, it's broken
into 2 × 800m instead of 4 × 400m. I then bring my recovery on.
I got the recovery time for my 800s down to 30 seconds and then

15, and finally I'd try and do four laps around 1 mile and come in at 6 minutes 25 or below. After six to eight weeks of building up to this, constantly looking at my watch to make sure that I'm hitting the pace and rhythm that I want, I start trying to do the reps without wearing my watch and have people time me so that I'm running on feeling. I then add more reps until I'm able to do 12 × 400m reps at my goal race pace without a watch and with minimal recovery (12 × 400m being 4800m, just 200m shy of 5k or a little under 3 miles).

That was the dream. And now the reality. You take what you learn at or on the track and apply it to longer distances and road runs. Even if you haven't got a track, you can mark or map out these distances in a park or around your block or local neighbourhood.

If you haven't got a race coming up, set your own goal by timing your 4 × 400m run and aim to improve on it – for example, if you average 100 seconds every 400m then aim to improve it to 99 seconds, and keep on working. I promise you will love the mental and physical feeling of nearing and then hitting your goal. Then you can move on to the next one.

Run at race pace

When people are training for races, they go out on race pace runs and a track is a brilliant place to do this. They calculate the speed at which they need to be running to achieve a certain time for an upcoming race – like I did for my 5k race, above, for my track work-out – and go for it. They want their body to get used to how a pace feels. They want to know what their body does, what the perfect leg turnover and arm drive feels like, how far they can push the pace before their body says NOPE, we have gone too far.

Race pace runs have kept me very honest. You can wish and hope and pray for times, but if you haven't put in the work the body will let you know fairly quickly. I went on a race pace run which was supposed to be 10 miles, but 6–7 miles in I was *dead, finished, frazzled, fried*. That let me know that I had a decision to make, I could either risk going out too hard, at a pace that my body had

Race pace runs have kept me very honest.

just told me was too fast, or I could slow down a little bit and still get a Personal Best. It wasn't what I had trained for but a few weeks off with a niggle had clearly done more damage than I'd thought.

It's the body's equivalent of putting a car into cruise control, or switching on the autopilot on a plane. The body is so used to it, it simply does what it remembers, what you have told it to do many times before. But just like any supercomputer, you must first programme the body or it has nothing to work from, and this is all about programming.

All of this helps you gauge your effort, based on several factors. And with time, practice, experience – and a little bit of luck – that gauge will become your friend and confidant. That gauge will be able to tell you what sort of pace you are running at and give you an idea of how much longer you can maintain such a pace.

But first you must be patient and get to know and understand your body, what it does and how it reacts to different paces.

Learn to run on feeling

Learning to run on feeling around the track is a great way to get better as a runner. You are essentially getting to know yourself and your body, getting to know what certain paces feel like, what your breathing sounds like, what it sounds like when your feet hit the ground. You start to read all the messages and signals that your body sends you and you're able to act on them in real time at any pace. After a while I genuinely felt like a little metronomic robot flying around our oval office.

One of the training sessions we did was to run 10–16 × 400m. We had a board set up at the side of the track. You had to pick a time that you'd run each 400m at and you could only be 2 seconds either side of your chosen time. So if you said you were running 75-second 400s you'd have to run each 400m in 73, 74, 75, 76 or 77 seconds. If you missed your time your rep didn't count. After a while we managed to do it, then we dropped it down to 1 second either side. The thing is, the longer you go the harder you have to work and the deeper you have to dig to maintain the time, so it's all about remembering where you put the effort in. I would always remember I kick off fairly quickly, accelerating round the first bend, easing off around the second bend, floating then pushing down the straight, easing off just a little on the third bend, then starting to build momentum again and kicking off the last bend pushing to the line. I'd remember what the wind felt like, how much my arms were pumping, how long I'd been running for. If I was running with other people I'd even remember what they sounded like. It's so weird to think of the things the human mind and body are made to do.

Tempo runs

After these intervals, speed or track workouts come tempo runs. Tempo runs are classed as comfortably challenging, verging on uncomfortable runs that build up to last between 20 and 60 minutes, or 5 and 10k. They are an important building block when trying to improve your fitness, endurance and strength. These runs help to improve your ability to manage discomfort for longer periods of time.

A great way to start to introduce a tempo run into your training would be a negative split run, which is a fancy way of saying finish the second half quicker than you did the first. Go out on a 20-minute run, do the first 10 minutes at an easy pace then pick it up to a comfortably hard pace that you know you can just about hold on to for 10 minutes. The aim is to eventually be able to run that pace for the full 20 minutes. If you find that that's too much, try doing 15 minutes, then 5 minutes, and work to a negative split. As time passes, you'll feel your body getting used to the pacing, so slowly start to change the times. Now try doing 8 minutes easy and 12 minutes hard, then 5 minutes easy and 15 minutes hard, until you can do the full 20 minutes. Then build more and try and do 10 minutes easy, 20 minutes hard, and repeat the exercise till you hit 30 minutes hard.

As time passes, you'll feel your body getting used to the pacing.

This doesn't happen overnight and will take time, gradually building. But isn't that half the fun, being able to watch yourself grow as a runner and as a person? Meanwhile, all the physical work is also helping to make you and your mind tougher and stronger. This is what happened to me and many others around me. We started standing taller, smiling bigger and hugging harder.

I have to say tempo runs are my favourite type of run as it's just beautiful. For me it's the closest I come to flying on my feet. It's when it all comes together and you are running at a pace that a few months previously was very, very uncomfortable to run at for even a short period of time. Now here you are at that same pace and going for double the time. It's like finding the sweet spot in third gear in a car – the engine is dancing in the powerband, if you push a little bit more the engine starts to scream and wants to change gear, so you keep it right here.

We used to run together through the Royal Parks or along the Embankment 10 to 20 deep, all of us dancing in our own sweet spot. No one speaking, all you could hear was breathing and the sound of our feet hitting the ground, until I'd raise my hand and scream 'TEMPOOOOOOO!' as we'd pick it up for the final push. The aim was to replicate a kick for the finish line, either to chase down someone leading, run away from someone chasing or trying to dip at the line to beat a PB. Visualisation always helped, regardless of what group I was with. Sometimes RDC or RDCWest, sometimes Nike Run Club, Good Gym or TrackMafia. The company may have been different but the goal remained the same.

Tempo runs are ideal training prep for a hard 5k or 10k, and also act as great building blocks for longer runs likes half marathons and marathons. Even though you'll be running at a slower pace for the longer distances, the fact that you have trained to manage the discomfort that comes with the tempo run will mean you'll be able to last longer in the uncomfortable place on a longer run. As I said, it's all building blocks or pieces of a puzzle that fit together.

Hills and hill repeats

After tempo runs come running up hills and hill repeats, which involve picking running routes that have lots of uphills and downhills. The reason you put in work on hills is because they double up as sneaky speed and run-specific strength workouts – driving up that hill is very good for strengthening the muscles you use for running. Hills are also great for building endurance – if you can power up a hill, imagine what you can do on a flat. Hill repeats are short, sharp uphills that help to build good running form and running efficiency.

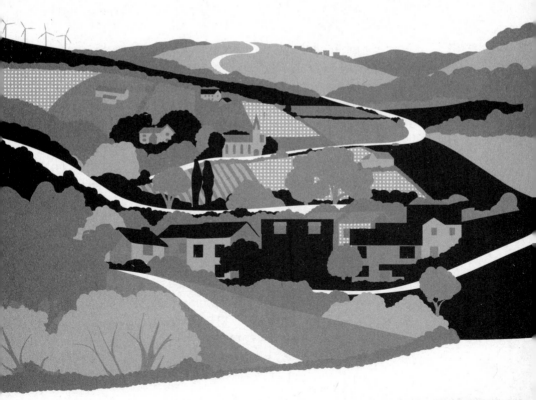

I started off by picking a small hill in Dulwich only 20 metres or so in height with a gradient of 4–6 per cent, and I would just do 5–10 reps. At first I started off at a really steady pace as I physically couldn't go any faster. After a few sessions on said hill I was able to go a little faster and didn't milk the recovery as much as I had done previously. But I had to take my time; with all things come a risk of injury, but especially with hill reps. If not managed correctly you could tweak your calves, quads or hamstrings – don't be like me, take your time and be patient.

After you've got used to the reps and the pace, you can drive up the hills a little quicker, find another longer hill and do the same. Once you get used to this, start incorporating hills into your runs. Or plan runs which are loops that take in long hills. The aim is to climb the hill and push off the top of it, NOT REST WHEN YOU GET TO THE TOP.

This is something that Coach Babs taught me. She told me not to rest at the top but to dig deeper, fly harder and use the brow of the hill as a launchpad to pick up the pace – it was not a place for rest and recovery.

We would do loops incorporating London Hampstead Heath's Swains Lane of Pain, as it is often referred to. It's a hill that's between 800m and 1km long, depending on where you start, and the incline averages around 8 per cent and peaks at 20 per cent, building its steepness as you progress further up, teasing and taunting you. (A gradient of 0–10 per cent is flat to moderate; 10–15 per cent is a little steeper; 15–20 per cent is pretty steep; 20–25 per cent is steep. Over 25 per cent is VERY STEEP. The max gradient of any climb in the world is between 34 and 36 per cent.) This hill was in no way fun or pleasant but Babs made it our playground. She

The aim is to climb the hill and push off the top of it.

suggested we train on this hill every weekend so that we could eventually do ten runs up and down, which meant 10 miles of hills. She called this routine Flatline.

The whole point of Flatline was to test your resolve, which would in turn help make you a tougher, stronger runner. I remember these hills really made a difference. Before, I would die running up hills in races and in other training runs people would either drop me on the hill, or I'd be able to hold on at an incline but at the top I'd fade. After training on these hills I was like a new man come race day. It's so rewarding – on hills that I had previously struggled up I was now bouncing, bounding, dancing up and flying over the brow.

They say that variety is the spice of life. The same applies to all these different types of runs. Variety can help to spice things up, fend off boredom and prevent you plateauing. I like to think of them as Lego bricks, every piece helps to make the building feel a little more secure. So try them out, start incorporating them in your runs. But take your time and work at a pace that you're comfortable with.

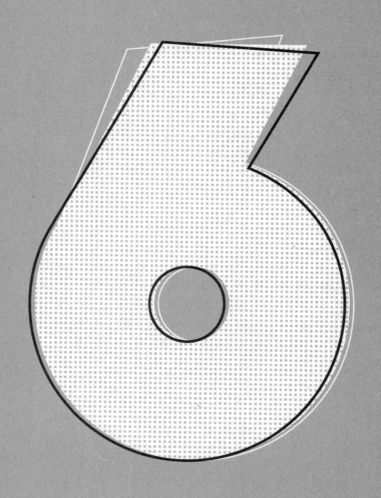

Set Goals

What's your destination?

A question that I get asked a lot as a runner and a coach, especially by beginners, is: how do I know what pace I should be running at? And the answer is, if you just started running, you don't. That's all part of the journey, something you must now explore. Running is very much like a game of chess, in that it's strategic whether you are running by yourself or are racing. You must think ahead and be willing to take a few risks, some calculated, some not. It's *allll* a game.

A great way to kickstart this game is honestly to just go out and run. As we saw in the previous chapter, whatever pace, speed or stride you naturally fall into will more than likely be your easy pace, and this is the pace that you should spend most of your time at when you are starting out. It's the pace that if you needed to you would be able to have a conversation at, so if you're not shy try talking while you run – and if you can't, ease off your pace. If the talk test isn't for you, try breathing through your nose instead of your mouth while you are running easy. If you're struggling to get enough air in through your nose, bring it down a notch.

When I first started I am not afraid or embarrassed to tell you that my easy pace hovered between 13 and 14 minute miles . . . I was a plodder, a steamboat that just chugged along. There were days when I ran a little faster and there were definitely days that I ran slower. The goal was always to be consistent regardless of the pace, which is what I want you to always have in the back of your mind. Consistency is key to both progression, belief in oneself and, weirdly enough, bulletproofing your body to help prevent injury. Your running pace isn't given, it's earned, and if you don't work to keep it once it's earned, it will be taken away by the running gods until such a time that they see fit to return it to you.

You will find that as time passes that easy pace becomes easier, so you start to pick up the pace without even realising and this new pace is now your easy pace. In my case my pace increased to somewhere between 11 and 12 minute miles after a month to six weeks of running. You will also find that there will be days when that easy pace feels harder, so you bring it down. It's all about how you and your body are feeling that day in that moment, and it's about the time or distance that you are running for. You will find that a sustainable pace is different over different distances.

If I told you to run to the bottom of the road as fast as you can, it would be a completely different pace to the pace you would run at if I asked you to run as fast as you can around your block, estate or complex – so bear that in mind. Also bear in mind that those paces may change based on a number of variables. They could be dependent on time of day, temperature, hydration, elevation, terrain, whether you are running on a flat, uphill, downhill, or whether you know the route or not.

Once you start to explore running a little more, a great way to help you set your goals is to predict your potential paces for distances like 5k, 10k, half marathon – even a marathon. Go out and run a mile as hard and as fast as you can. Either map out the route with no traffic lights or do it in a park, or on the track. Once you have your all-out mile pace, you can tap into all sorts of fancy mathematical algorithms that people way smarter than me have put together.

These are commonly referred to as race pace calculators – you can find tons of them online. These tools are pretty accurate but may not predict the fighting spirit that we are sometimes able to tap into when the going gets tough. Just to be clear though, it's doubtful that that fighting spirit will make you run 1 or 2 minutes faster per mile, I'm talking about a few seconds.

Now I had the numbers I actually had to do the maths, not with my brain but WITH MY BODY.

After I'd decided I wanted to start running, but before I actually started, I reckoned I wanted to achieve these things: I wanted to run a sub 30-minute 5k, a sub 60-minute 10k, a sub 2-hour half marathon and finally a sub 4-hour marathon. At that time I don't think I had wised up yet – no Bronze, Silver or Gold times. Just numbers.

I didn't think these were huge goals. I remember thinking that all of these things would be hard, but they'd be achievable at some point before I died. I mean, how hard could it be, right?

I'm not quite sure where these goals came from. Presumably from friends and random readings on the Net, illogical internal debate followed up with yet more guesswork. Without having any experience, and determined to aim for something, I fixed on these goals and set to it. Thing is, now I had the numbers I actually had to do the maths, not with my brain but WITH MY BODY.

To put it simply, if you *physically* can't run a 5k in under 30 minutes it's unlikely – not impossible, but *very* unlikely – that at the same level of fitness you would be able to run 10k in under 60 minutes. The same applies if you can't run a half marathon in under 2 hours; if so it's unlikely you can bang out a sub 4-hour marathon. I'm sure somewhere there are exceptions to this rule, but I for sure was not one of them.

As I write I remember my first proper 5k. I was thinking to myself, dude, dude, *duuuuuuuuude*, how the hell are you going to finish this? How on earth are you in this much pain, this much discomfort, for this little itty-bitty race, how are you going to do this eight times over with a little sprint at the end? That race had taken me well over 30 minutes and it wasn't as if I hadn't tried. I crossed that finish line *spent* . . . huffing and puffing as if I chain smoked hundreds of cigarettes a day.

At the time I felt proud that I had finished but I was secretly unhappy that I hadn't come in under 30 minutes as I had planned to. That feeling passed as I realised that there would be other days, other times to try and get in under 30 minutes.

The same thing happened to me over the 10k distance. I remember *battling* with my body, first just to be able to run for 60 minutes without stopping for a cheeky break and then to be able to cover 10k in under 60 minutes.

When I first started trying to cover the 10k distance I plotted the route out so I knew exactly where I was going and how far I was at nearly every point in the run. I would always get through around 80 or 90 per cent of the distance and then I'd give up mentally. I would find a reason to slow down or stop or find an excuse as to why today wasn't the day. One day I thought, hmmmmm, I wonder if changing the route might work? Changing the route to one that I wasn't so familiar with, one that wasn't tainted with what I referred to as my failures (a word that has since been upgraded to learnings). So change the route I did and miraculously it worked. I had no idea how long I had been running or the pace, as I didn't look at my watch, and the only reason I kinda knew how far I had gone was because I was getting closer to my house. The goal for that day was to simply enjoy the run and embrace the unexpected. It worked. A few weeks later I went back to my old route to exorcise those demons and once again it worked.

Now that I could cover the distance without stopping it was time to take it to the races.

In the beginning it was always the age-old thing of things were going so well until they weren't. I remember trying out a number of different racing techniques. First I tried going out all guns blazing then trying to hold on after banking time. *Ha*. Foolish, foolish idea on my part as I just ended up walking large parts of it after killing off my legs and lungs. I tried going out easy and easing into it, but ended up crossing the line feeling like I could have gone harder and longer.

This taught me yet another lesson about running and life. And that is: it's one distance but there are so many ways to approach it. Some may say there's a right way or a wrong way, but I would add a little caveat to that and that is there's a right way for some that might be wrong for others.

What I hadn't realised is that though at the time this running thing felt like a fruitless task, it was teaching me things, giving me lessons that I may not have learnt otherwise. Running taught me to be far more patient, far more confident and courageous. Forgiving, courteous, understanding, able to meet challenges face on, to understand that if meeting challenges face on wasn't working there was another way. It taught me more about problem solving and thinking in the moment than any course I've taken or job I've had. WHY? Because I always have skin in the game, as they say, it's always me and my body on the line. Every single last one of these lessons benefited my life outside of running. I think the biggest takeaway from running was definitely my confidence. I was far more willing to put myself out there and not so worried about not getting something right. Running gave me my smile back, it made me happy.

Every time I stopped short of what I wanted to achieve I was actually learning valuable lessons for my next attempt. And every time I ran – faster, slow, long or short – I gave my body more experience and muscle memory for the next run. Any time I failed to meet a speed goal I was still strengthening my body with fitness and stamina.

Now we've all been on some kind of course or read something about setting SMART GOALS. We have to make sure that the goal we set is:

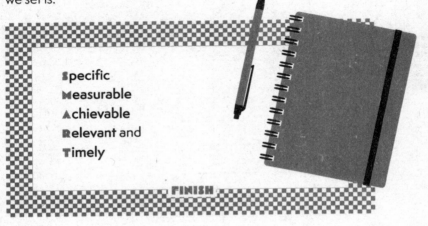

Specific
Measurable
Achievable
Relevant and
Timely

FINISH

All the goals I was setting myself were specific, they were measurable and they were achievable, but in the time that I had given myself they were completely *unrealistic* – mine were not SMART goals . . . They were neither relevant nor timely.

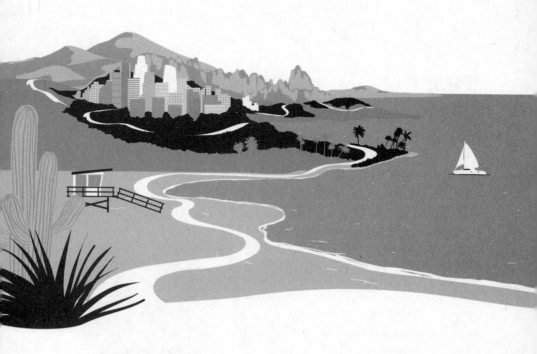

Specific

Specific goals help you stay motivated as you have something to either look forward to or work towards. That goal needs to be exactly what you say it is, specific not general, and a great way to get to that goal is to ask yourself, WHAT DO I WANT TO ACCOMPLISH? A general goal might be 'I would like to run faster than I have ever run before'. To make that specific you might change it to 'I want to beat my PB or PR by 2 minutes'. Or if it's distance based: I want to cover 100 metres more in x amount of time. If you are just getting into running, your specific goal might be to sign up for a 1 mile race or 5k on a specific date.

Measurable

Having a way to make those specific goals **measurable** is important, but equally, so is allowing yourself to make adjustments to those goals if things aren't going to plan. A great way to get to that goal is to ask yourself HOW FAR? Or HOW LONG? And then HOW WILL I KNOW when I have done it? The end goal could be to run 5k in three months. In order to reach that goal, you would follow a plan setting out certain distances that needed to be run on certain days. It could be as simple as run three times a week, Monday, Wednesday and Friday, and every week the time or distance goes up. This would make it feel like you had lots of little goals leading up to the big goal and your celebration. Something that I love about running. I say this as I find it hard to think about things way, way in advance, which is why I have even more respect for Olympians and other world-class athletes who always seem to be thinking four years ahead. As a side note, it's quite hard to measure, but outside of racing, one of my goals has always been to *enjoy* my running. Even if I don't smile right that second in the moment, I measure many of my runs by how big a smile I have on my face or what kind of mood I'm in when I am finished. Unless I got injured or things went really, really wrong, I can't remember a time when I felt worse about myself after a good run.

Achievable

The goals you set should be **achievable**, and not unrealistic like the goals that I set myself very early on in my running life. Ask yourself: what do I need to do to accomplish this goal? How will I get there? And what are the things that could stop me? Set goals that sit just outside your comfort zone but not so far that they are unattainable, as that can negatively impact you and your running. Instead of feeling like the hero that you are, you end up feeling like you have failed or let yourself down. So ask yourself, based on what you know, do you have the time to train for the goal that you have set yourself? Are you willing to put in the work to reach your goal? And do you have everything that you need to set yourself up for success? If the answer is YES, YES, YES, you are off to a better start than I was. If the answer is a *hmmm* or a no, fear not, you have plenty of time to adjust your goal. And that is the beauty of this. YOU ARE IN CONTROL.

Relevant

When I say your goal should be **relevant**, I mean it should be something that you think is both worthwhile and important. Something that's meaningful and personal to you.

This should help drive you. When I ran my first few races it was to prove to myself and others that I could do it. It was also about raising money for charity. Then it was about losing weight and getting fitter, then it was my mental health, mourning and therapy, then it was to make friends, to explore the world, then it was using running as a tool to help with my creative process. As I said before, it was the gift that just kept on giving. So ask yourself, what gift are you looking for? Not anyone else, YOU.

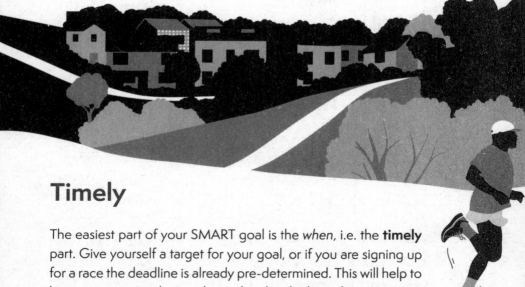

Timely

The easiest part of your SMART goal is the *when*, i.e. the **timely** part. Give yourself a target for your goal, or if you are signing up for a race the deadline is already pre-determined. This will help to keep you motivated as you know that the clock is ticking. Knowing that you have a deadline will also motivate you to keep working, as you know that you have invested time, money and yourself. But remember what I said before: don't be afraid to shift the goal posts if you know that for whatever reason the goal is no longer realistic. Hold yourself accountable, but *don't* beat yourself up about it. Find out why things didn't go to plan and work on being better next time, as we are *allllll* a work in progress.

I remember looking into training way back in the beginning, but the training I was looking into was training for a marathon and it just so happens that I would do a 5k, 10k and half marathon on the way.

Based on the maths, in order for me to achieve the beautiful sub 4-hour marathon I wanted, I would have to be able to run a sub 1:50 half marathon at 8:47 minutes per mile pacing, a sub 50-minute 10k at 8:24 mile pacing and a 5k in under 25 minutes. I would have had to be running around 20 miles a week already and that distance would have had to be done over three or four days. So, you see, from the get-go I set myself up for a result that I didn't want.

My advice to anyone, whether you are just starting out or you have been running forever is that if you have a goal that is time based, be honest with yourself and do the maths. It doesn't have always have to be surgical, but it should be SMART. If you are going for a time, you can only get to that time if you work towards it. Don't just pluck numbers from the sky and hope and pray that things will work out.

Back then it took me 33–34 minutes to run a 5k, 68–72 minutes to run a 10k and over 2½ hours to run a half marathon and well, my first marathon took me nearly 7 hours, as I've already told you.

Don't just pluck numbers from the sky and hope and pray that things will work out.

Seven hours of struggle and strain, seven hours of life-changing goodness that at the time I struggled to deal with.

Looking back on things now, the biggest mistake I made was the one that changed my life. I signed up for a marathon and ran that marathon a year later. From a purely running point of view, if I was going to do it again – and if I was prepared to sacrifice all the mental benefits and growth I got from doing it the way I did – I would change everything. No way would I do a marathon after a year. I would drop some weight and spend a lot longer building my base endurance. Then I would work on speed over shorter distances. A tempo pace over longer distances or in between my longer runs, and technique for shorter distances. All of this comes together and helps you to up your pace and improve your speed endurance, which helps you and your body deal with the demands of longer distances. I would say I had the potential to become a baby bullet train, but instead I became a long-distance coal powered steam train that just kept going . . . but not quickly.

Here are a few goals to think about, regardless of where you are on your running journey:

>> Walk fast.
>> Run for the first time.
>> Run to the bottom of the road without stopping.
>> Run around the block without stopping.
>> Clock your first, fastest or fabulously fun km.
>> Clock your first, fastest or fabulously fun mile.
>> Enjoy your run, and smile while you are doing it.
>> Clock your first 2 miles.
>> Clock your first 5k.
>> Do a parkrun.
>> Clock your first 10k.
>> Enter a race at any of the aforementioned distances and set yourself a Bronze, Silver and Gold time. And remember to celebrate regardless of what happens.
>> Do all of that again and celebrate how far you have come – remember, time isn't the only way to measure progression. Did you feel better? Did you smile more? Is it easier to climb that set of stairs or get out of that chair?
>> Remember to SMILE.

Do all of the above and share your world with someone else. Give the gift of running to a friend, loved one or work colleague.

I've saved this one till last as that's what I did. When I first started running, unbeknown to myself, I inspired my mum, Lyn, and little sister, Janeen, to begin running, too. Watching them run and go through what I did brings so much joy to my heart . . . it's the gift that keeps on giving.

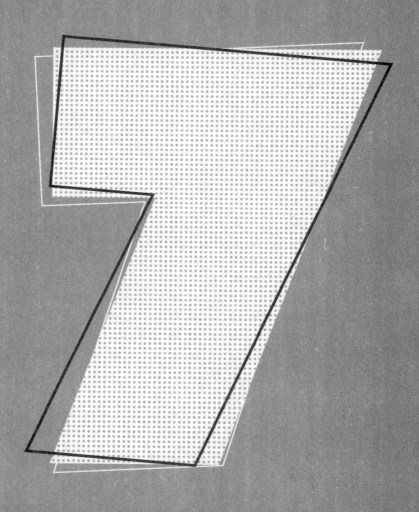

The Toll It Takes

How to deal with injuries

've had so many injuries, and most of them, if I'm honest, could have been prevented had I really listened to my body and done all the work that I should have done. Some injuries are avoidable as they stem from overuse or doing too much too soon, and others seem to be part and parcel of running. In the early days I appeared to be a magnet for many of them, I felt like I was being unfairly targeted by them, which is something I hear a lot when speaking to runners. It's something that can make you or break you.

Part of the problem is that beginners to running, or to sport in general, find it very hard to identify whether something is painful due to an injury or simply to a lack of readiness and fitness. My advice is LISTEN TO YOUR BODY and if in doubt STOP. I frequently made the same mistake of powering through discomfort when what I should have done is STOP.

I'll tell you about some of the most common running injuries, what kind of pain to expect, what's serious, what to do and what not to do. But ultimately you are the captain of your ship, and as time passes you will learn all the ins and outs of that ship and get better and better at recognising what's what and making more informed decisions. It's like with anything new, it takes time.

Fear not though. Many common injuries just need rest, ice, sleep, good nutrition and a few days off. Others may stop you running for a few weeks or months. But don't be disheartened; just give your-self time to heal, time to recover, and you'll get yourself back out there. These are injuries that many runners suffer and they won't stop you running forever. You'll need to do the stretches, work on mobility, build the strength and understand that it's a journey and you are always a WORK IN PROGRESS. Some take a break of 1–2 weeks, some 2–4, some 1–3 months, but in all my years of running, people tend be back after most common injuries in a few weeks to a month.

In the first couple of months I picked up many of the injuries runners get either when they first start or when they are trying to build mileage or time on their feet. I'll touch on my experiences with them: injuries such as plantar fasciitis, runner's knee, iliotibial band (ITB) syndrome, Achilles tendonitis and shin splints, as well as strains or pulls of muscles like the calf or hamstring, and a few other worthwhile mentions that are more annoyances than injuries.

Before we really get into this, I want to be real clear up front: these are *my* experiences, things that have happened to me, and how I and the people I have dealt with have treated them. If you have an injury, go and get it seen to before it gets worse. I am not a doctor, surgeon, physio or health professional, I am just a runner who's been beaten up by the road and trails and have somehow made it to a laptop to share some of my highs and lows with you. So I say again: if you're hurt, or think something is up, GO SEE SOMEONE. ☻

Plantar fasciitis

The first thing I noticed a few weeks after starting running was an annoying nagging *hummmmmm*, a shooting pain in the soles of my feet right near the arch, gradually working its way to my heel and back. Not just in one, but in both feet at the same time, although it seemed to be worse in my right foot. It was as if my feet were trying to clench into a fist without my permission and it would come on suddenly, this squeezing feeling. I'd feel warm strings of pain running along the bottom of my feet, all of them being pulled at the same time so that they felt tight and cramped. The pain could be excruciating and it would come while I was running, sometimes a few minutes after I started running and sometimes when I was a lot longer into a run. Sometimes I felt it as soon as I woke up in the morning.

If I was on a run, I'd have to really slow down or stretch the soles of my feet by taking my shoes off and pressing down through my toes or pulling my toes towards me. If I slowed down I'd have to completely change the way that I ran; it turned into more of a hobble than a run.

It really hurt. It hurt physically to the point where I'd be on the verge of crying, because it was painful but also frustrating. I started to question myself and my confidence dwindled. I didn't know what I was dealing with, I thought I could run through the pain and hoped it would sort itself out. This was wrong of course, because you can't run through plantar fasciitis, which is what this was.

Plantar fasciitis is one the most common running injuries. It's the inflammation of the **plantar fascia**. What's the plantar fascia, I hear you cry? That's the magic stuff or strong connective tissue that runs *alllllll* the way along the bottom of your feet from heel to toe. It can get inflamed and painful when you suddenly do a lot more walking or running, or exercise with a tight calf or heel. You can help to prevent this from happening by stretching and strengthening the soles of your feet and calves. As well as by breaking up the fascia on the soles of your feet.

To help break up the fascia on the soles of my feet I have regular foot massages. When I can't get to the masseuse for whatever reason I use a small massage ball or spongy hockey ball that I roll underneath my feet, I apply a little bit of pressure to the areas where I am feeling the most tension, aka the trigger point, but not too much pressure as if you do it too much you do more damage to your feet. This is called **self-myofascial release**, or SMR for short. Don't be fooled by the long words, it's a fancy way of saying 'I massaged myself'. Try doing this not only before and after runs but also if you're sat at your desk. But as I said, not too much and not too hard.

To this day, my plantar fasciitis will still rear its ugly head from time to time if I don't do all the things that I'm supposed to do. STRETCH, STRENGTHEN, REST AND MASSAGE. And if it does, I treat it the same way I did before. I haven't had it really bad since the early days, but when I did, I would freeze a small bottle of water and when I woke up and my feet were really tight, I'd roll the bottle underneath. I'd also place a towel on the floor and try to pick it up with my toes. This also helps to loosen up the fascia. When I got bored doing that, I'd use the same towel to wrap around my toes so I could pull them towards me for a stretch.

Fallen arches or flat feet

I have low arches – or flat feet – which commonly leads to plantar fasciitis, as it did for me. Coach Babs recommended that I strengthen my arches by doing heel raises. It's exactly what it sounds like.

You start with your feet flat on the floor and raise your heels while putting your weight on the balls of your feet. It's as if someone slipped some heels on you then slipped them off. I'd start off by doing both heels at the same time, 3–8 at a time, then build from there. Once I was strong enough to do that I tried single legs, just doing 2–5 at time.

Picking up marbles or anything small and round from the floor, or scrunching a towel between your toes and releasing it is also great for strengthening your arches. After a good three to six months of doing exercises like this every day the plantar fasciitis agony was no more on long runs. But the moment I stopped doing them, it came back. It taught me a valuable lesson. They work if you work.

FINISH

Blisters and battered toenails

Blisters, as well as battered, broken black toenails, are more of annoyance than an injury but they can still end a race or slow you down.

Just like many other runners, I'd get blisters a lot when I first started as my skin was still very soft and I was yet to develop that tough layer of rhino skin that I needed to prevent my poor sock and shoe choices from ravaging my feet. I'd get blisters on the arches of my feet, on the heels and in between my toes. Some would bubble up and burst and some would be bloody. And yes, yes, yes, blisters are painful, and I'd feel them with every stride, but after a while I stopped getting them.

You can limit the chances of getting blisters by wearing shoes that are the right size for you and wearing proper running socks that will wick away the sweat as you move. If you know you have softer skin and are prone to blisters, there are special patches or plasters that you can buy to help prevent you from getting them. I'm not saying that they will always work, but they are there to be tried and tested.

The same applies for the aforementioned black toenails, often caused by shoes that are too small or – guess what? – too big. Your feet either move around too much and smash against the front of the toe box of your shoe, or your shoes are too tight and your toes smash against the front of the toe box of your shoe. Both culminating in the same thing: UNNECESSARY PAIN.

Now, I am sure you can see a pattern developing that would suggest that getting the right type of shoe, a shoe that fits correctly, *and* matching it with a sock that wicks away sweat, would be a good idea when you start to up the mileage. Or why not start as you mean to go on and invest early *if you can*. If this toe boxing, toe banging happens repeatedly your toenail will go black and fall off . . . and then . . . you wait for it to grow back. THE END lol.

I know this, *oooooh*, too well and all from personal experience, or from friends that I've been running with for years. There was a point and time where I honestly had more toes without toenails than toes *with* toenails. For a while, open-toe sandals were side-stepped in favour of shoes that would hide what lay beneath as I waited for the nails to grow back. And, yes, they have all grown back beautifully. They are now regularly looked after by my local nail technician – PEDICURES ARE A MUST.

There was a point and time where I honestly had more toes without toenails than toes *with* toenails.

Did I run without toenails? Of course I did, unless it was painful to do so – and even then I'd just stick a little plaster on top and off I went.

Just to be clear, it's normal to lose a few toenails here or there in running circles. DO NOT PANIC. If it happens to you, they will return, they will just take their time.

And sometimes, the toenails that grow back are even more beautiful than the ones that have been left behind.

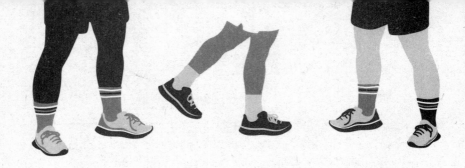

Rolled ankles

As if I didn't have enough to worry about with my feet in the early days, I rolled my ankle a few times. Sometimes I would be running and place my feet badly, either on a paving slab that would move without warning, on a tree root that was hiding from me, or on something else that was in my way. I wasn't used to reacting quickly to things like that, so my ankles would roll out away from or in towards my body and I'd strain or overstretch the ligaments that supported them. On some occasions I'd just wince and carry on and the following day the ankle would be swollen. I'd ice it, rest it until the swelling went down and the pain was gone, and get back to work.

On some occasions I'd just wince and carry on and the following day the ankle would be swollen.

On other occasions I'd roll it and be out for weeks, sometimes months. The little injury had become a big injury because I'd continued to run on it when what I should have done was put myself in a cab, which may have meant less time spent recovering. I'd also come back too soon and because the ankle wasn't fully repaired it was more susceptible to being rolled again. The first few times I was in panic mode, so I went to the hospital or doctor and had it looked at, but the more I got used to running and injuries the more I realised that there are many things that you just know as a runner, like how long this injury is going to keep me off the road due to swelling and level of mobility. And when you don't know you go and see a physio.

The longest I was out with a rolled ankle was a few months. I was running a leg at a 24-hour trail race called TR24. I was running downhill at night in the pouring rain through thick mud, when I took a sidestep to avoid another runner who had cleverly stopped in the middle of the course on the brow of a hill. And that was that. My foot got caught in the mud and rolled outwards, and as the medical staff said, 'I'm surprised it's not broken.' Thank goodness it wasn't.

After lots of rest and once the pain had subsided, I had to do lots of rehab on my ankle to strengthen the surrounding muscles and tendons that supported it. This is also the kind of work that can prevent your ankle from rolling in the first place.

It's like I was retraining how my ankle should behave if I was put in a similar situation. I did a lot of exercises to work on my ankles' proprioception, aka how they react naturally to terrain when my body is on autopilot – exercises on one leg that focused on BALANCE and STRENGTH. Standing on one leg while catching or throwing a ball, or standing on an uneven surface, wobble ball, board or bosu ball. I'd brush my teeth on one leg, stand at the bus stop or wait for coffee on one leg. The idea was to get my ankle used to making more adjustments on my behalf. And it worked. Of course I still roll my ankles from time to time, like any runner does. But the reaction and recovery is definitely quicker.

Shin splints

Shin splints were the next present that running gifted me. Shin splints is the term used to describe pain along the shin bone, the big bone in the front of your lower leg.

Shin splints can rear their ugly heads because of poor running form, fatigue from doing too much too soon, not running in supportive enough footwear or running in footwear that's too supportive for the way that you run. If your shoes or innersoles are too supportive or too corrective they can prevent your body's natural suspension from doing what it's designed to do.

The first time I experienced them I had no idea what was going on. It was as if somehow I had slapped a large piece of bread to the side of my shin and that piece of bread was now part of me. Not only was it part of me but it also seemed to have a heartbeat every time I took a stride, painfully pulsing and causing me real discomfort. At the time I didn't even know I could feel pain there.

I treated that with plenty of rest, self-massage, stretching, lots of ice, a few anti-inflammatories to bring the swelling down and a smarter approach to increasing my mileage. The self-massage and stretching helped, but what *really* helped long term was getting stronger and working on my mobility. Also paying more attention to my running form, making sure I was standing tall when I ran, landing beneath my mass, pumping my arms and looking straight ahead with a nice long spine. These are little tweaks you can make to help improve your running form.

Calf injuries

After the shins came the calf injuries, something that has haunted me from the beginning. I would be out running and I'd feel my calves tightening, making it harder to run. Sometimes the pain was just on the surface, but most of the time the pain went deeper into my calf, deep into a muscle called the **soleus**.

As it was mild discomfort rather than a shooting pain, I thought it was just fatigue. If I had rested the way I should have done, eaten what I should, strengthened and worked on my mobility the way I should have, it would have just been fatigue. Instead, it became an injury.

According to a bunch of studies, every stride you take when running you put anywhere between 1.5 and 8 times your body weight through your legs and, dependent on how you run, the brunt of that weight will go through your calves. This means that if you haven't prepared them properly by either starting out slow or doing a proper warm-up, they won't be happy. It was especially true for me because at the time I not only had underdeveloped calves, but I was also overweight and had poor running form, so my calves were really getting hit.

There were times when I'd be out of action for a few days with a little niggle, times I'd be out for a few weeks. Other times I'd be out for months, slowly, slowly trying to come back but then coming back too soon. And when I say too soon, I mean there were times when it would hurt to walk but I'd try and run anyway because I really wanted to get back to it. There were other times when I was ready to run but I should have gone easy, avoiding running fast and hills, sticking to steady runs with single and double calf raises to help strengthen them so it wouldn't happen again. Both instances resulted in longer healing times.

If you get calf pain: STOP and REST, take it easy and don't push it like I did.

If you get calf pain: STOP and REST, take it easy and don't push it like I did. If it does become an injury, do the usual rest and ice. Stretching isn't advised unless it's ADVISED BY A PROFESSIONAL because it can do more damage than good, so try using a foam roller on your calves and regular massage. And don't go back out there until you're properly recovered.

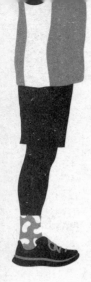

Iliotibial band pain

After my calves came pain in my iliotibial band, or ITB as it is more commonly known. It's a thick band of tissue that runs along the outside of your thigh, starting at your hip bone and ending around the top of your shinbone. The pain comes from friction where the ITB crosses over your knee.

My ITB would flare up or get annoyed with me when I ran too much and didn't rest enough, when I ran too fast or increased my mileage too quickly and didn't rest enough or attacked hills. And guess what? I didn't rest enough. My ITB would hurt as there was a lot of friction where it crossed over my knee. This would cause swelling if I didn't foam roll it, massage gun it, have it massaged, stretch it, warm it, or cool down properly. So don't be like me. Do all the things I just said I didn't to help prevent you from experiencing the discomfort I and many others have had to go through.

If your ITB does become inflamed and overworked it tends to feel like a warm achy burn, or it may feel very sore and tender around your knee as well, with a similar pain up and down the outside of your leg.

Hamstring strains

After my ITB came my hamstrings, which would go *ping*, *ping*, *ping* if I ran too fast for too long or too soon after I started running. They'd also go *ping* if I overstretched them, hadn't stretched them enough or had overworked them doing hill repeats and hadn't given them enough time to recover. Most of the time it was my fault for pushing too hard, but on the odd occasion I would be running and be surprised by a shooting pain. It would feel as if someone had stabbed me with a little knife, then when I touched the area a little later it would feel tight like a little knot was there. I'd have it strapped with tape or a compression sleeve and just like everything else I'd follow the path to recovery. And so can you: RICE (Rest-Ice-Compression-Elevation), pain management and anti-inflammatories if it's not too bad; seek out a medical professional if it is. Only you will know where the line is, but don't push that line out too far to save money or be a hero. You only have one body . . . LOOK AFTER IT.

Tight quads

I have never injured my quads, but I *do* have to stretch them a lot. If I don't they get way too tight. When they get way too tight it can cause my pelvis to tilt, which then puts a lot of pressure on my lower back. So sometimes my back would hurt but the cause of it would be from tight quads, so I'd stretch, stretch, stretch and foam roll the life out of them. I advise you to keep on top of that.

Tight back

The same applies to the lower back. I've never had a back injury but I *have* had tightness around my back, because my core wasn't strong enough and it got tired keeping my body upright for miles and miles. So my core sent a signal out saying I'M WEAK, I NEED HELP, and like the good teammate my lower back is he came charging in on his horse and then him and his horse got tired leading to my back pain. To think, all of this could have been prevented if I'd stretched my quads and worked more on my core. Just added a few exercises to my daily routine. Exercises like planks of all variations, Russian twists, glute bridges, single-leg glute bridges, crunches, sit-ups, mountain climbers – all of which can be done at home. Or some yoga or Pilates. I suggest you work on your core. Why? A strong core is what keeps you upright, it helps with posture and alignment.

And that helps you to run faster and staves off injuries, it's what helps your upper body and lower body work effortlessly together. The stronger your core, the less strain the rest of your body will suffer with every stride you take.

Chafing and bleeding nipples

I can't talk about injuries, inconveniences and annoyances and not mention chafing, a running annoyance that I am more than familiar with.

Chafing tends to happen when you're running and either skin rubs on skin or skin rubs on clothing creating friction. I, as well as many others, have experienced said chafing on my thighs, especially the inner thigh area, my armpits – and my favourite place, nipples. There are two incidents I'll never forget.

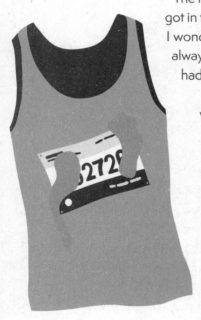

The first time, I never knew I had nipple chafing until I got in the shower and screamed as the water hit them. I wondered what the gods was going on. They were always a little sensitive, but I didn't realise all the skin had been rubbed off them by my running T-shirt.

My second favourite incident happened when I ran a half marathon in a white vest – the Stockholm Half, I believe it was. It was fool-ish of me to run in a tight white singlet with no protection for my nipples. I was in the zone, just concentrating on ticking off the miles. I got to Cheer Dem Crew, a cheering station that had been set up around mile 10 of the 13.1, and all I heard was ARE YOU OK? I screamed back 'Yes – water please!' They said 'Yes, but are you OK?' I said why, and they said 'Your nipples are bleeding!' I looked down and my vest was *bloody*. I smiled and kept on running.

Next time I used more Vaseline and made sure my clothing wasn't too tight and not too loose as PREVENTION IS BETTER THAN CURE. I could have also got myself nipple guards or nipple protectors – yes, they are absolutely a thing – but ample Vaseline seems to work for me.

And to treat my poor nipples: warm salt water and some antiseptic cream. Lesson learned.

Tension in the upper body

The upper body is something that we tend to forget about, as it's our legs that carry us. *But* something to be mindful about is the amount of tension that we carry up there if as runners we don't work on our mobility and range of motion through stretching, yoga, massage, foam rolling, etc. That tension can cause pain in your shoulders, upper back, and neck muscles. All of that can prevent you from moving as freely as you'd like when you run and even cause headaches. Whenever I go and see my masseuse or physio, they always laugh and ask: 'Why do your shoulders feel like bricks? Why do you have so many knots in your back?' In the beginning, when I'd say it's all from running, they'd say no way and get to work. As time has passed, I have definitely got better at looking after myself, and so can you. Make sure you give your upper body a workout – stretch, lift weights, do core work (see Chapter 4). It all helps to keep you free and limber when you run.

began to take my training more seriously when I started to work with Coach Babs. She asked me what kind of things I wanted to get out of working with her. I said I wanted her to make me 'injury proof'. She laughed. I asked, 'Why are you laughing?' She said, 'When you say "injury proof" what do you mean? Can you define it for me?' I said, 'I want you to train me, so I get to a place where I just don't get injured, or at least not a long-term injury.'

She laughed even louder and said, 'When you say a long-term injury, what do you mean? What do you class as long term?' I said, 'Anything that keeps me out of running for longer than say three weeks is classed as a long-term injury to me. Well, a month, tops.' The thought of not being able to run or train for something for that many weeks seemed like a long time.

She continued to laugh. She said, 'Cory, first, there are professional athletes as well as normal everyday people just like you who have been out injured for as little as a few months and as much as a few years and are still trying to make their return to full fitness and running.

'There are people who have been cross-training and strengthening their bodies in preparation to come back once their bodies allow. I can't make you injury proof; anyone that tells you that they can is lying. We can work on things that will bring the chance of you injuring yourself down, like strengthening your body and mind, working on your weight, nutrition, recovery, mobility, flexibility, more sleep, running form, etc. But sadly, when you get to a place where you are pushing your body, it's pretty hard to avoid any kind of injury.'

I sighed and said, '*Ah*, so like everything else, my fate will be left to the gods – let's just do what we can then.' So that we did.

The more I worked with Babs, and the more I ran, read, watched, listened and learned, the more I realised that running, staying fit and injury free is like spinning a wheel. It's one big experiment with a sprinkling of luck. An experiment with your body. A balancing act – the art of finding the crucial combination of getting enough nutrition, sleep, rest and recovery while pushing your body to a place where it doesn't want to be. A place of discomfort but not pain. A place where that discomfort is embraced and your body changes, so that the next time or the time after that, the discomfort comes a little bit later as you now have the ability to push harder earlier.

But to get there, a calculated risk must be taken – to get there you must be consistent, it's one of the biggest tools that can be used for injury prevention. It's the routine of running that gets your body ready to do it again and again. So, weird as it sounds, CONSISTENCY IS KEY to getting your body used to putting in work. It is key to your body developing and growing to support this love of yours.

The biggest injury I've had has been to my left knee. I saw everything that I'd worked for so hard and so long disappearing off into the distance and I'm still not 100 per cent sure of how I managed to do it. I was even more annoyed as prior to that, I'd never had any problems with it.

I was at Paddington Recreation Ground, the home track of TrackMafia. I had finished work early so I went downstairs to get a good session in. I honestly can't fully remember the session after the warm-up and drills but it was a speed session involving lots of hard 200m followed by plyometric exercises, both single leg and double leg (a posh way of me saying I jumped around a little). Plyometric exercises are a form of exercise that uses fast, powerful movements to help improve speed, strength, power and sometimes balance and endurance, depending on the exercise. Other examples of this are skipping, bounding, jumping rope, hopping, lunges, jump squats and box jumps.

I finished the session and noticed that my left knee felt weird. Really tight and swollen. I phoned Babs and said something was up. I tried to run but I didn't seem to be able to run at the pace I was at before. She asked me to try and do a few moves, so I did, and we worked out that if I could do A and B then it wouldn't be C. She said, 'See how it is in the morning.'

I woke up in the morning and *panicked* as my knee was now the size of my head. I went to see Babs straight away at her Energy Lab Studio, but we still couldn't work out what it was – we just knew it wasn't my anterior cruciate ligament (ACL), the ligament in the middle of the knee that's commonly injured in sports. I went to see another physio and a doctor and their tests couldn't confirm what it was either. I was still able to run, just not fast, and I had trouble running around corners quickly.

It was recommended that I rest and stay off the knee. I said, 'That's great advice, but this is my life and on this occasion rest isn't going to fix it.' I was starting to get scared as this mystery injury was essentially threatening my running and career. The question is, how do you fix a problem when you don't know what it is? You research all that you can and seek help from everywhere you can.

So I did just that. I spoke with Emmanuel Ovola, aka Manni, a friend of mine and a member of TrackMafia who was not only a runner but also a physio. He referred me to a knee specialist who he felt would be able to help me and for that I will always be grateful, so here in black and white I thank you again, Manni.

I went and had tests done, and initially the doc was just as bemused as everyone else until he asked me to do a single-leg squat. He looked at me and said the body is a wonderful thing. 'Can you see what your leg is doing? We'll get you in for some scans but it looks like you've torn your meniscus' – the little c-shaped pad of cartilage in your knee that acts as a shock absorber – 'and if you want to continue to do what you do at the level that you want to do it, you're more than likely going to have to have keyhole surgery on your knee.' I just looked at him and, shall we say, I got a little emotional. I was happy that I now knew what the problem was, *but* I had also confirmed that it was a big problem. I'd confirmed that I needed surgery, I'd confirmed that I had actually hurt myself for real this time and just rest wouldn't cut it.

Injury is part and parcel of running, it's how you deal with injury that will make or break you.

I left the hospital and phoned Jules crying. She calmed me down and said it would all be okay. I phoned Babs crying; she said it would all be okay too, and as I'm writing this I'm crying, as when I heard the words come out the doc's mouth I really didn't think that everything was going to be okay. The thing is, running was my way out of unhappiness, a way into a new way of life, and this injury was threatening it.

But I had to pull myself together. Of course I gave myself time to be sad, to try and deal with the emotion. But as Babs had said to me all those years before, injury is part and parcel of running, it's how you deal with injury that will make or break you.

I went back to the hospital and had the scan and the doctor confirmed that my meniscus was severely banged up, but he said that once they got in there, did the surgery and cleaned it up I shouldn't have any more problems. He said I could have the surgery as soon as a few weeks or as far away as a few months. When would I like to have it? I said I'd consult with my coach and come back.

On speaking to Babs, she said I'd recover more quickly if I did Prehab – aka Preparation for Rehabilitation – so that I'd get a head start on the rehab. She said, 'Why not take the time to strengthen all the muscles that surround and support the knee to help you come back stronger? Why not push the surgery back as far as you can. You can still run at a steady pace, cycle, row, squat and all the other things. And if you do all of those things as planned we will turn you into QUADZILLA, so the knee has ample support post-surgery.' So we did just that. QUADZILLA is what I became.

I let the surgeon know that I'd like to push my surgery back by six to nine months, the longest I could, so that I could get to work. He gave me the nod, and a date, and from then, I cycled every-where to build my legs. I ran at a steady pace, I lost weight so that it would be less of strain on my knee. I tweaked my diet, I slept more, I did everything in my power to be ready for this surgery and when it came time, READY I WAS. I had a successful keyhole surgery and did everything that I was told to do by both my surgeon and my Babs, and a few months after that surgery I ran my fastest marathon. I'm telling you this long drawn-out story with all these twists and turns because I want you to know that when you are injured you can and will go through the whole spectrum of emotions. Sadness, anger, regret. You'll blame yourself, blame others, blame the road, the track, the trails. *But* when it's all said and done, you have to BE HONEST – you have to DO THE WORK – you have to TAKE RESPONSIBILITY. Or there will be no comeback – or, worse yet, you won't even find out what's really holding you back.

I couldn't have done this alone. You have to surround yourself with people who have got your back, people who will support you. So thank you to everyone who helped me come back, but especially my surgeon and Manni for their care and wise words, Babs for beasting me and showing me the way, and Jules who held my hand at every step. Seeing them both cheering me on as I came steaming through mile 22 at the London Marathon was a very special moment for me. It made me feel like regardless of what happens, I'll always dig deep. And that's all you can ever ask of yourself, not just when you're injured or hurting but in life – NEVER GIVE UP.

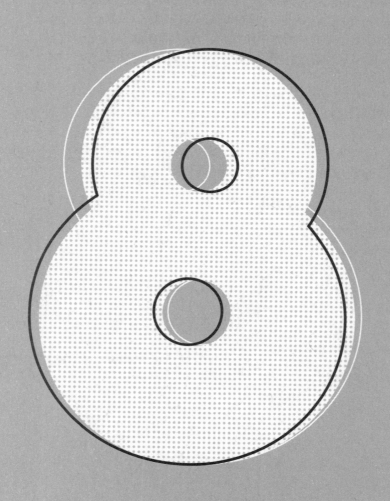

Time
for an
Adventure

Where can you run?

When I first started putting one foot in front of the other, I had no idea that running was actually a passport that unlocked the world. Running gives you a reason to explore and it took me to places that I had never really thought about visiting. It also gave me an opportunity in many cases to explore them like a local as opposed to a tourist.

I will happily hold my hand up and say that, prior to starting to run, I had no idea how many races there were, how frequently they happened, how many different terrains you could run on, how many distances were run and – most importantly – how many people of all shapes, sizes and ages ran. I am not saying that I thought the only race in the world was the London Marathon, but it was the only one on my radar.

I later found out that you can literally run a race every day of the year over a number of distances if you really want to. *And* there weren't just road races, you could also enter:

» Races run virtually on a treadmill.
» Off-road races that take you through the countryside or parks in major cities.
» Trail races that take you through the woods and forests, up mountains and across li'l streams and maybe even a lake.
» Races on beaches through the sand or in the desert.
» Races on the track, even if you aren't a professional runner.
» Cross-country leagues that you can join with a running club.
» And of course, my favourite type of race, a race where the route is run through a number of mixed terrains. You might start off in the woods, run on the road then finish up on the track.
» And we can't forget races through the snow.

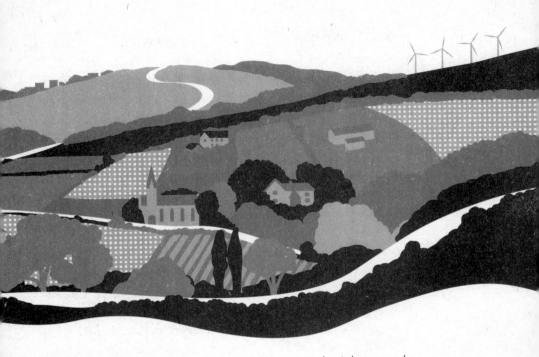

On top of all of this, there are races that you don't have to do alone. If you wanted to do one with friends for the social aspect, or you just wanted to break up the distance, you could run the race as a team, like a relay. Or there are races that set up to *only* be run as a team, whether they are from point A to point B, or whether as a team you might have 24 hours to do as many laps of a set course as you can.

My mind was blown by the many other weird and wonderful things that could be done with running. I had no plan, I just dove in, ran what was available, loved it and learned from it. At the time I had no idea how valuable all these races were to me, how much knowledge I was picking up, and how blessed I was to be in a position where I could go to all of these places now that I had a body that was willing go where I took it and do what I asked it to do. Albeit a little slower than I'd liked. (I smiled as typed that.)

There are a bunch of places that you can find out about races now, but at the time there were only a few. I would find them on the Runner's World website in the events section. You could enter the dates, location and distance you were looking for and it would give you a list of races. You could either pay there directly or it would push you to another website to enter. For some you would get confirmation of your entry and then something in the post, and for others you would have to turn up with your ID in hand and they would give you your racing bib and safety pins then.

As it was just me, I had no one else to please, so I would go online and look for random obscure races in places that were anywhere from ten minutes' to three hours' drive away, fill up my car with petrol and off I'd go to a village that I'd never heard of, or a town I'd never been to, bright and breezy on a Saturday or Sunday. I would head out to places like Epping, Richmond, Sutton, Caterham, Brighton, Guildford, Windsor, Reading, Oxford, Derby, Southend, Bournemouth and occasionally as far afield as Wales.

More often than not I was the only Black dude there and quite often one of the only bigger-bodied dudes there.

More often than not I was the only Black dude there and quite often one of the only bigger-bodied dudes there. People were always very welcoming and supportive, but I was very aware that it was just me out there. I didn't really mind, but I did wonder. Where are all the black folk? When I look at the TV a majority of the people in the long-distance races look like me, albeit smaller and slimmer, so where were they? And yes, I know that many of the runners are running for countries like Ethiopia, Kenya and Uganda, and this is Britain – but I still wondered. Where was my representation? I thought, OK, so it's not there, then

I will have to represent. It's weird that you even have to think like that, but you do. In a space where you are the only one or one of the few, you have to be bold, lead with your chest and wave that flag of yours with pride.

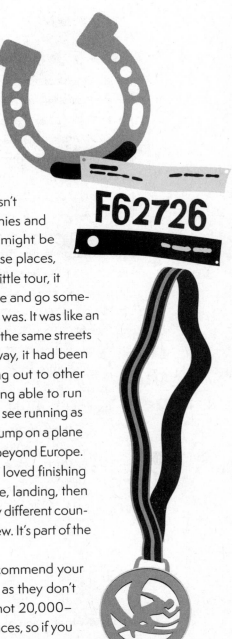

At that point, *anywhere* outside of London felt like it was far, far away and I wasn't sure why I loved heading out to the boonies and running these races. But now, I think it might be because I had never been to most of those places, and it gave me an opportunity to have a little tour, it gave me a chance to get out of my routine and go somewhere different where no one knew who I was. It was like an adventure. For someone who had walked the same streets all their life, and who grew up a certain way, it had been easy to fall into the thinking that pushing out to other places was just for other people, but being able to run broke me out of that. And to this day, I still see running as an opportunity to go on an adventure. To jump on a plane and explore other places beyond the UK, beyond Europe. It's not an excuse to travel, it's a reason. I loved finishing coaching at the track, jumping on a plane, landing, then coaching on another track in a completely different country or running with friends both old and new. It's part of the culture and now part of me.

If you are just starting out, I would recommend your first race being a small countryside race as they don't have a huge field of people. There are not 20,000–30,000 people to navigate like the big races, so if you are concerned about being intimidated, feeling anxious or lost in the crowd, it's perfect. Some races will have fewer than 100 people, some 100–500 and even more all the way up till you get to the really big races I mentioned earlier. These smaller races will either be through woods, a park, or along a canal towpath or roads. For some of the races the roads will be closed while on others you will have to navigate open roads with the assistance of marshals. Some will have chip timing (in which a microchip attached to your running bib or number registers the exact time you cross the start and finish lines), at others it will be volunteers with stopwatches. And as the runners don't set off in a series of big waves, everyone starts at the same time so your time will start as soon as the gun goes off, and when you finish you might be ushered into a line so they don't lose where you came in the race.

The beauty of these smaller races is that because they have small fields, you might find yourself placing and winning a cash prize, voucher or trophy. For some races there will be medals, at others you'll get a pat on the back and a thank you, and at yet other races you get a belt buckle or horseshoe as your medal.

These races vary in length from short distances like 1 mile all the way up to a half marathon, and some are 20-mile races that have been set up specifically to help people who are training for marathons. The beauty of the different types of terrain is they all offer something a little different.

Treadmill

Running on the treadmill is great, especially in places where the weather acts as a barrier – you might be in Montreal in the winter when it's too cold to run or in Qatar in the summer when it's too hot. The treadmill has the answer. I am speaking from experience: I remember a time a few years back when I was out in Qatar with Jason, aka NotAfraidToFail, who's a good friend of mine and an amazing photographer.

He was photographing the World Athletics Championships and I was there with Nike creating content in my role as European head coach, riding camels in the desert and sharing my views on the races with the world. I needed to get a run in as I was training for my next bout of ridiculousness, so I was dressed and ready to head out. I thought, 'It's early, it won't be too bad.'

Maaaaate, the moment that door open I was struck by a wall of heat that I felt I wouldn't survive, so I took myself upstairs and hit the treadmill. The treadmill gave me consistency, a little less impact on my legs, and I was able to pick the pace that I wanted to run at then switch it up when I wanted to do intervals. I brought the incline up when I wanted to smash some hills and I was able to jump off when the legs started to feel a little sleepy or I wanted to recover. The treadmill is a great tool for runners of all levels; I used it when I started and I still use it now. If you've never used one, hit the gym one day and give it a whirl.

Don't get me wrong, when I get the chance to be outside I love to hit the trails or do a bit of cross-country running. I find running outside to be a more engaging experience, with all that fresh air, trees, wildlife and people watching. But when it's not available I can appreciate group classes on a treadmill, either led in person by a coach or virtually via a recording or app like Fitness+.

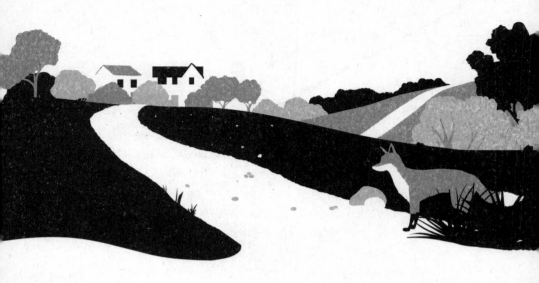

Trail running

Trail running is all about getting off the road and into NATURE. Trail runs feel like a lot more work than running on a flat road or on the treadmill. The reason they feel harder is because they are. A lot of the time the terrain and surface that you are running on will change, there could be lots of sneaky uphills or inclines that help to build a little more strength in your legs. You have to be a lot more aware of your surroundings, so you have to use your eyes and engage your brain a little more. I love how that extra challenge can feel like a game. It's harder to switch on autopilot and just cruise – you have to look out for tree stumps, rocks, roots, branches and, of course, wild-life. Combine that with the uneven surface and you are working on switching up your stride length constantly, increasing the strength in your ankles, improving your running ABCs: Agility, Balance and Coordination – *and* your proprioception. As we've seen, the official meaning of proprioception is your body's ability to sense move-ment, action and location. This is useful when running as it helps to prevent injury, making you less likely to roll your ankle due to a greater awareness of your surroundings and increased responsive-ness to said surroundings.

I have run some amazing trail races and trained on some amazing trails. My favourite race was definitely the Trail Wales half marathon out in Coed y Brenin Forest Park in Snowdonia. It was probably one of the toughest races I have done. I remember literally clawing my way up a hill as I definitely couldn't run up it. I tried walking up it but the technical incline had other plans for me, so I ended up having to put my hands into the mud – so you could say I *crawled* with a beautiful backdrop in a trail-running paradise.

Old school cross-country

If you can't get out to trail-running paradise, why not take it back to school and try out some old-school cross-country running, a race that is either run in teams or as an individual. Cross-country – known often as XC – is typically run over dirt or grass either in a park or in the countryside, and often includes hills, flats, minor natural obstacles and maybe even some water; the courses vary in length from 2.5 to 7.5 miles. Living in London most of my life, XC was always run in awful weather conditions like rain, sleet, snow or hail, which made it – get this – *even more fun*. For those of you *blesssssed* with better, or I'd rather say 'different' weather . . . I may have envied you as I ran head on into hail and wind.

Living in London most of my life, XC was always run in awful weather conditions like rain, sleet, snow or hail.

A few years after running that magical trail race, I was invited out to a rural town in Ethiopia called Bekoji to work with a charity called the Girls Gotta Run Foundation, who invest in young female change-makers through education and running. A friend of mine, Knox, was working on a documentary and asked if I would like to come along and capture some behind-the-scenes footage, do some good and train under the watchful eye of the legend that is coach Sintayehu in a place that is often referred to as the 'Town of Runners'. This dude is the coach who worked on honing the talents of the likes of athletes like Tirunesh Dibaba and Kenenisa Bekele, who at the time were Olympic and World Champion middle-distance runners.

It really was something special to be out there running in the motherland, training with people who lived and breathed running. My first visit was an eye-opener as Bekoji sits 10,500 feet above sea level. That means every breath you take has around 33 per cent less oxygen in it. This makes things a lot harder; it's as if someone splits your lungs in three and says, okay, you only have access to two-thirds of your lungs for the duration of your stay. Now go train with the pros or those trying to make it as pros.

My first few days were tough but special, and I learnt so much. My biggest take-away from the trip was USE YOUR ENVIRONMENT as much as you can. We spent a lot of time in the woods and we would pick up branches and spread them out evenly in the grass, using them as markers for drills and for hurdles. Coach Sintayehu would purposely pick routes through the woods that were hilly and technical to help build strength. We would zigzag through trees working on our speed, agility, balance and coordination, and all of the running drills would be done in unison to build team spirit and unity. This helped me look at the trails and woods differently. It made me realise that, of course, equipment is nice, but Mother Nature has provided us with everything that we need to become stronger, more efficient runners. All we have to do is think outside the box, realising what's been there since time began. If that doesn't work, either make your own box or create a shape of your own, which is the route that I had decided to take long ago.

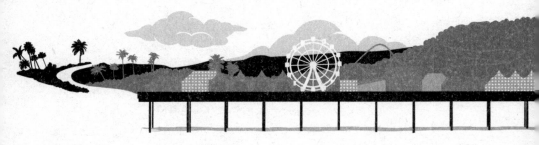

Create some fun

Many years ago I realised that running was pretty boring. Yes, I said it. I loved it, but I *knew* that it was boring to many people. I also knew that many people would find running a little more fun and engaging if someone could make it a little more interesting. So I tried to do just that.

It started off in Westminster at Paddington Recreation Ground with something called Oyster Monday. I was running a group with Ellie Wood called RunDemCrewWest, the baby sister group to Charlie Dark's RunDemCrew, which was based out in Shoreditch. I realised that we could run further if we didn't have to run out and back. Instead, we would run out then get the train back using our Oyster cards. On the way back on the train we would do a body weight workout – push-ups, dips, squats, etc. – and commuters would cheer us on. While running I would point out places of interest like palaces, museums, lakes, statues, sneaker stores, coffee shops or restaurants that I thought were cool. I noticed that many people either hadn't been to or hadn't heard of many of the places that I was pointing out. So I thought, why not make a race or challenge out of this, as people seem to be happy to run if they have a real reason.

After that I sat down with a notepad and plotted out my first proper event. It was called Mission Impossible, and the idea was that people could enter in teams of two to four and would have three hours to try and run to as many locations as they could and take a picture. I had T-shirts made, medals, stickers, trophies, and hired out a small bar in

Shoreditch to host it. It was here that I really started to use the phrase LEAVE IT ON THE ROAD, a phrase that meant so many things to me. It was like a nice way of saying 'all guts and glory' combined with 'be kind to yourself', as each run would be different. Regardless, the task was the same: LEAVE IT ON THE ROAD. Give the road what it's asking for and leave it all out there: your feelings, your emotions, any doubt that you have. The idea is that running offers you more than just a run if you need it, so use it, take advantage of it and the road will reward you.

I was blown away by how many people offered to help, by how many people turned up and how much fun it was. I couldn't have done it without all the volunteers who showed up on the day and the support from my running community and family. But a special shout out needs to go to Darren Sumpter, Chop aka Mark Fleming, Ellie Wood, Charlie Dark and Eugene Minogue. Without them I wouldn't have even got the ball rolling. After that I really got a taste for organising random events that I felt would engage a different type of runner, or help people who weren't into running get into it.

Give the road what it's asking for and leave it all out there: your feelings, your emotions, any doubt that you have.

Next up was something called TellNoOne. The idea was to completely go against what everyone else was doing. I only invited people whose phone numbers I had and no social media was allowed before, during or directly after the event. The events would always start off late at night, somewhere between 10 p.m. and midnight. We would meet in a bar called Shutterbug in Shoreditch (it was run by our friend Cathy – hello Cathy!). I prepared a document that gave the rules of engagement – all written very cryptically and placed in envelopes. We would snack and have a few soft drinks then I would hand out the envelopes. They would open them and read:

> *Pick a partner and plot a route.*
> *You have 60 mins to cross the River Thames as many times as you can using different bridges.*
> *You must run through two royal parks, past two museums and take a picture with someone wearing a suit and someone who works for Transport for London.*
> *There are no losers, only winners; the first team back wins.*
> *You leave in 60 seconds.*
> *Now, RUN!*

The point was to get people to use the streets like a playground and use their bodies to explore it by night, so some people would run 5k, others 10 to 15k, and some days we would all run together. Want to try it?

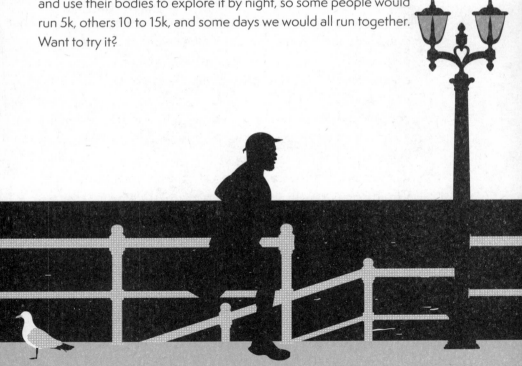

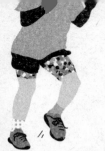
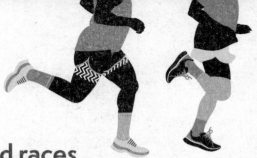

Run clubs and races

The beauty of running together or as a relay team is you get to cover distances that you may not have been able to cover alone, and having teammates that depend on you makes you push a little harder.

After reading all of this you might be asking yourself, as a beginner runner, if I'm just starting out, when is the best time to join a running club? Based on my own experience, if I was starting from the beginning all over again and was thinking about joining a running club, I would wait until I could run for a mile without stopping or two miles with stops at traffic lights.

I'd work my way up to this distance by myself or with friends, or with the help of apps or virtual coaching, and I would ideally do it outside, as opposed to on a treadmill, before joining a run club, *unless* the club specifically says they are open to beginners – perhaps a club that describes themselves as a beginners' group, or a couch to 5k group. I say this as I think it's easier to set yourself up to win and feel good about running. It's great to have aspirational people in the distance and say to yourself 'I'll get there one day', but if they are too fast, or too far away, it can leave you feeling like you're in the wrong place, you're not fit enough or fast enough. When that's simply not the case – you're just not ready for that group yet. Which is fine. You can work your way towards that. So my advice is to join a club as and when you feel ready and when they are ready for you. Then prepare to be exposed to all the wonderful leagues and relay races, community and camaraderie.

My first experience of this sense of community was in a race called the Welsh Castle Relay with the first running club I joined, Dulwich Runners. I had seen this club out running in Sydenham and Crystal Palace; they always flew past me on the hills that I was dying on. I did a little research on the club on the old World Wide Web and found out that they were open to beginners and their main club night was on Wednesday evenings at 7.15 p.m. Runs varied in length from 5k to 16k or 3 miles to 10 miles and varied in pace from 5-minute miling up to 12-minute miling. They were founded back in 1980 and they were still going, so I thought they must be doing something right. I'm happy I was right.

The Welsh Castle Relay is a two-day, 20-stage, 209-mile *staggered* relay stage race, organised by Les Croupiers Running Club Cardiff and held mostly on road but with a ton of hills and mountains en route from Caernarfon to Cardiff, with a cheeky overnight stay in Newtown. The race is staggered so each stage starts at a particular time, regardless of whether or not the last person has finished the last leg. The legs vary from 7 miles to 13.1 miles and on each team there are ten people, so you run one leg each day and act as support for the rest of time. Those that are supporting are in one of two vans. One van waits for the runner to finish and picks them up, the other has already gone ahead and dropped off the next runner. Now you may ask, is this a race for a beginner? I would say it's a great race for a beginner to work towards with a mixed group. Do I wish I'd done this race or races like this when I first started? HELL YES. If only I knew, I would have had something even more fun and exciting to work towards.

Join a club as and when you feel ready and when they are ready for you.

Another race like that which isn't as hilly and which I also did with Dulwich Runners is called the Green Belt Relay, which is a 22-stage running relay around 220 miles of the Green Belt around the outside of London over a single weekend, organised by the Stragglers running club. Kicking off at Hampton Court and finishing in Bushy Park, the course mainly follows footpaths, towpaths and minor roads and involves around 50 teams of eleven, who each run one leg on both days. Although the race is a relay, each stage starts at a fixed time, just like the Welsh Castle Relay. This means that each stage can be a competitive race in its own right if people so wish. Rumour has it that founder Sean Davis has walked every inch of the 220 miles and visited every church, castle, windmill and lockkeeper's cottage along the way.

I loved running both of these races, as it showed a different side to running that I had no idea existed. I experienced it with an old-school running club wearing their colours, and I spent the whole weekend on both races smiling ear to ear as I felt like part of a team who were trying to achieve something. I was slow but no one cared. All they cared about was that I was giving my all.

If you like the sound of relay races like this but you want something that's continuous, you can find races like that too. My first continuous relay, the TR24 race I mentioned in Chapter 7, was held out in the countryside. The course is 10k in length and is packed full of different trails, challenges and terrains. As you probably guessed

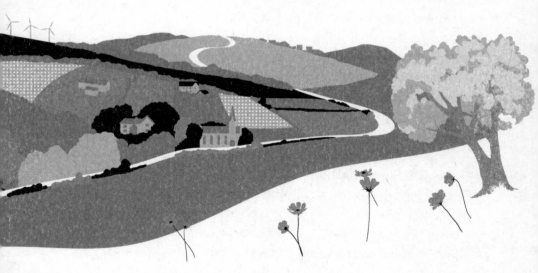

from the name, you run for 24 hours in total. You can run it solo, in pairs, or in teams of three to five or six to eight. You get to run in the day, the night and then the day again, so you get to see the sun set and then rise which is a beautiful, beautiful rewarding thing. You take turns to run either one lap at a time or more, and wait for your turn to come round again. While you're waiting, you're either cheering, eating, preparing food for someone else to eat or you're sleeping in the tent that you set up earlier in preparation for your next run. It was the first time I had ever run while camping and I must say it was a blast. You can imagine the energy coming from all the tents and all the teams. It's like a mini festival – they have stalls cooking and selling food through the night, as well as drinks for the participants and special drinks for those who just came to cheer.

Being in one place as we all ran one lap was amazing, but once again I wanted to try something different, so while visiting the Nike World Headquarters in Portland, Oregon, myself and some friends took on a race called the Hood to Coast, a relay that is often referred to – for good reason – as the Mother of All Relays. There are 36 stages that vary in length from 3.5 miles to about 7.5 miles, and you run in teams of eight to twelve for 199 miles from the top of Mount Hood in Portland to the beaches of the Pacific Ocean. Each team-mate runs three legs and though it sounds like a lot, I have taken a few beginners out to races like this. You get lots of support and, if managed properly, REST.

The beauty of this run is it's about more than running. You have to really work as a team to help and support each other. You split your team in two, half in one van and half in another. One van works and runs while the other one sleeps and prepares to be tagged in. You either sleep in the van, in between running your legs and cheering your teammates on, or in designated sleeping fields that come up later on in the race. You're running on open roads, so during the day we wear bright clothes and at night-time a high-vis vest, headlamps, and flashing lights on your back so you can be seen. I was super excited to run this race as I'd heard how epic it was. I mean, come on, how many races have sold out for 30 years straight? And it didn't disappoint, it was such an amazing experience. So much so I went back and volunteered as a photographer for a friend's team a few years later. And then took a group of young people out to the Netherlands to participate in the Dutch version, which was even more epic as I got to be there for a group who, like me, never knew this race existed. Then, as if I needed to travel a little more, I went out with a group of friends to Hood to Coast Taiwan to support, drive and photograph them running and living their best life. Big thank you to Edson and Joseph – like many things, without our random chance conversation over Thai food in our favourite Thai restaurant and a willingness to just explore, that would never have happened.

As we are talking about relays, I have one more for you . . . The Speed Project. As I mentioned in Chapter 4, I ran this race with friends a few years back. Nils, the founder, describes it as a gruelling 340-mile relay race that starts at the Santa Monica pier and ends at the Welcome to Las Vegas sign. There are no assigned legs, stages or distances. You just have to get from Los Angeles to Las Vegas in one piece. You can run solo, in a pair or in a big team, so the distance you run depends on you. We started off doing 10k each, then dropped to 5k each, then 3k each, then 1k each; then it's just do what you can and jump back in the van – running through

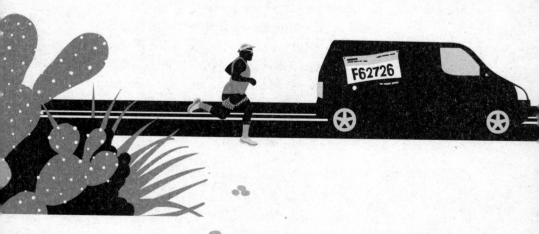

Death Valley in the middle of the day with temperatures in the 90s and 100s is FUN but NOT EASY.

When I first started running I didn't know any of this world existed – hundreds if not thousands of races in the UK and many thousands more around the world, all organised by people who live and breathe the sport. When I realised it was there I didn't just want to take, I wanted to give a little, which is one of the many reasons we started putting on races. And weirdly enough, whenever I think about putting on an event for people to run, I think of *what hasn't been done before*, not what has. I think of where we are *not supposed to run* and I work with friends to change that narrative. And it's these discussions with friends that allow you to activate running events in places like go-kart tracks, empty buildings, shopping centres and my favourite, football stadiums like Wembley Stadium.

You can run wherever you want . . . you just need to possess the will to do so. And if you have read this far . . . I believe YOU POSSESS THAT WILL.

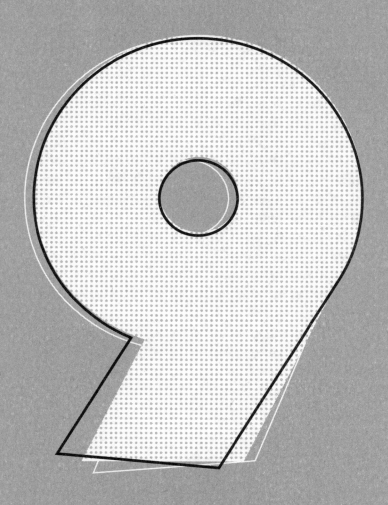

Find Your Family

Running is *community*

Community is about people you believe in, and people who believe in you. You are there for each other, you like a lot of the same things and are willing to learn about the things that others in your community want to share with you, even if it's not number one on your list. Community is about a mutual belief system, it's about caring and sharing. It's about trust, it's about taking from the well but most importantly it's about refilling the well. It's about a common understanding that we are all there for the greater good. Your community nurtures you, congratulates you, cares for you, supports when you need it, but also tells you when you've done wrong.

My running community, or my running *family*, mean everything to me. Without them I wouldn't have grown and discovered my true potential. Without them I would be in exactly the same place fighting the same demons, or maybe even being defeated by them. My running community truly built me up and helped me create the life I have now.

When I first started, I did it alone, as everyone else I knew that ran was either a seasoned runner or just *waaaaay* faster than me. Running by myself gave me life lessons. It taught me how to battle, how to struggle and how to dig a little bit deeper than I previously knew I could – or wanted to. My community, however, taught me how to love, which is a far more powerful tool, as you will do almost anything for the love of something. There will be times when you want to stop and give up, but for the sake of those that you love you will continue; you will push harder and go further and that's what I found.

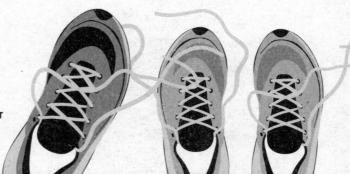

joined my first community, Dulwich Runners, years after I ran my first marathon, probably around 2009. I joined them for several reasons. I felt like I had plateaued in my marathon training, I had gone as fast as I could and as far as I wanted to without help and I thought I would learn a lot more from seasoned vets who had been there, done it and got the T-shirt. And luckily, it just so happened that I frequently saw these runners.

They were always polite and encouraging as they floated past me on a hill that I regularly did battle with, struggling to get to the top without stopping. It was a hill that I had named 'the wedding cake' – I called it that as it was tiered just like a wedding cake. It's around 1.5 miles long from bottom to top and isn't even that steep, it's just gradual, but for a newbie it's *unrelenting*. The first part is fairly flat, only around a 1 per cent incline, but the further you climb the steeper it gets. With 100 metres left to climb you're on anywhere between 9 and 12 per cent, which is easy for some but was way steep for me. Every time I tried to run up this thing I would gas myself out and have to walk, or I would be running so slowly people would stroll past me. I thought to myself: maybe they can help me conquer this thing as I'm clearly doing something wrong.

So, one day I bit the bullet. I searched for them online, contacted them via email and asked the question . . . *hey*, can I come out to play please? I didn't give them my running résumé, I simply said I had recently started running, I had a few marathons under my belt but I still knew nothing about running and gave them my running pace. 'Do you have a group that runs at that pace?' They came back to me and asked me to come on down.

I was invited to run with them a few times to get a feel for the club and see if it was the right fit for my needs. If it was for me, I could join the club officially and run for them in their colours. They had one main club night every week for everyone, and covered distances from 3 to 10 miles or 5 to 16k. There was a track night in the summer and weekend runs for those who were training for something. I said thanks, I'll see you soon.

Now I won't pretend like I packed my bag and rubbed my hands together thinking *yeaaaaaah*, can't wait to start. It was actually the complete opposite. I thought: *Ahhh* no, now I've committed to this I have to go. I've seen them run, they are fast, they have no body fat, they are going to laugh at me, and I am going to get lost. I'm not going to go. I am literally laughing out loud now as I remember how quickly my brain tried to shut this whole new thing down. How many of you reading this have experienced a similar feeling of dread when wanting to start something new? I want to let you know it's NORMAL and it's OKAY. But I also want to let you know that there are times when we have to make ourselves a little uncomfortable in order to grow. So that's what I did, I made myself uncomfortable. It was the best decision I could have made.

I rocked up wearing *faaaar* too many clothes. In my head I was dressed for a run in the cold and dark, but what I *actually* looked like was someone who was dressed to conceal his identity and wanted to get lost in the dark, dark nearby woods. They welcomed me with open arms, introduced me to my buddy for the evening who showed me the ropes, then off we went. I was *waaay waaaay waaaaay* at the back and even the steadiest pace was too fast for me, so as soon as we hit the hills I got dropped. They waited for me at the lights, then I got dropped again. I said, 'I'll see you back at the club as I don't want to mess up your run.'

When I got back to the club, they were waiting for me. There are a number of things that I could have done or said. I could have moaned that I was left behind, I could have said that I wasn't coming back as I could have got lost, I could have said that they were running too fast for a beginners group. But I said *none of that* because it was ON ME. Everything was on the website; it gave the pace they would run at, how long they would run for, what route they would take and

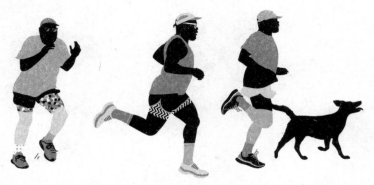

what hills were involved. And it was me who chose to go, and it was me who had to choose if I was going to go again.

My decision was simple: I'm going to keep going till I can hang with them. The little donkey now had a magical carrot dangling in front of him that he would devour before the year was out.

It was my commitment to getting better and my attitude that endeared me to them. I didn't care about coming last, I cared about the effort that I made, and so did my new friends. Dulwich Runners took me under their wing and took me to local races, cross-country meets, relay races, road trips. They invited me to socials, curry nights, picnics. They helped me discover a part of myself that I didn't even know was there. They showed me once again that it doesn't matter how old you are, where you are from or what your beliefs are. If you have running in common, I'm sure you'll have a bunch of other stuff in common too.

That was my introduction to my first running community. One that shall be referred to as the CLUB.

Next up came the CREW, or should I say RunDemCrew (RDC), the group of people that has had the biggest impact on my life, founded by teacher, DJ, poet and producer Charlie Dark many, many moons ago as an alternative to the running clubs that existed at the time. Based in Shoreditch at the then 1948 Nike Store, RDC offered something different to those that were looking for something different; emphasis was placed on the importance of looking after one another. Community, culture, fellowship, and the mentoring of young people

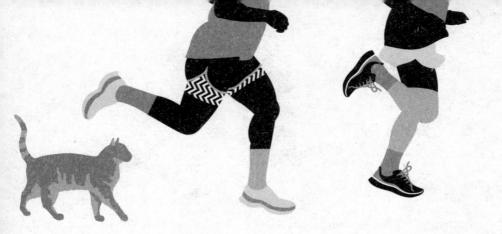

were at the forefront of the RunDemCrew running experience. It was more about people becoming better versions of themselves, using running as the tool or catalyst for that transformation, than it was about hitting times and qualifying for races. It was a social club where people hung out and people just so happened to be in running kit, running.

Now, to be totally clear before I go any further, I want to clarify that there may well have been other running clubs or organisations that existed on Planet Earth that put community and personal growth first and foremost, front and centre before running. But in my world, the spaces that I existed in, what I saw, what I felt, what I experienced, I hadn't seen or felt anything like this since school.

A few years after I started to take running just a little bit more seriously, I was introduced to Charlie Dark by Eugene. We were trying to get a parkrun off the ground at our facility, Paddington Recreation Ground in Westminster, but we just didn't seem to have the space that was needed. Charlie and Eugene had had discussions about setting up RunDemCrewWest to complement the offering over in Shoreditch. RDCWest was to act like an overflow for RDC, as the original weekly session was getting anywhere between 100 and 200 people every Tuesday.

The majority of the people who came had to write a letter to Charlie stating why they wanted to join the crew. Charlie would also send them a series of questions that they had to answer and if the answers clicked and balance could be found, you were in. If they didn't, you weren't – it was as simple as that. Balance was and still is one of the keys to success. Some may think it harsh but look at it this way: if you are inviting people onto your island, you want people who are going to help you prosper and grow, not people who will mash up the terrain and drain it of resources. It wasn't about your demographic, where you came from, how old you were or what you did, it was about your energy and why you were knocking on the door. I say this as crew members included everyone from dog walkers, artists, designers and schoolteachers to barristers, pilots and stunt riders.

Community, culture, fellowship, and the mentoring of young people were at the forefront of the RunDemCrew running experience.

Eugene set up the meeting where I met Charlie for the first time. I had obviously done some research, but I still had no idea who Charlie Dark really was or what a big deal it was to be sat talking with him. We discussed my running background, my running qualifications and my vision for the weekly session and my future. All of which have since changed.

What surprised me the most about our initial meet was that Charlie seemed far more interested in me, my background and my life outside of running, than he was in my running. We had quite a few things in common that led to deeper discussions: both raised as black men in deep South London by loving mothers, both spent time in private schools surrounded mostly by people that didn't look like us and both had a love for music. Especially music with a HEAVY HEAVY BASS LINE like reggae, jungle, and drum and bass.

I mention the time we'd spent at private schools surrounded by people who didn't look like us because with that knowledge we immediately had an unspoken bond. I went to an old-school private primary with rules that should have died out with the dinosaurs, so I was given the cane and the slipper for what now I would describe as minor indiscretions. I had no idea if Charlie had been caned in school, but I did know that we'd both experienced feelings of isolation and exclusion, whether intentional or not.

Of course, you can make friends and get on with anyone, but sadly at a young age you get to experience casual racism and micro-aggressions, which lead to a feeling of not belonging. And from a very young age you learn to *act*, to code switch, to take the bass out of your voice and make yourself small. You see your white friends treated differently, so you try and be more like them to fit in. That eats away at your identity and your feeling of worth. And even at a young age I was very vocal about not wanting to be there. But I didn't want to let my family down as I knew this school wasn't cheap. My mum was working so many jobs to keep me there and she sent my sister to private school as well because she wanted us to have the best. She knew how tough it was out there, so she wanted us to have a great education as a great education is supposed to lead to a better quality of life: you have the potential to earn more money and mix with people who are supposed to be heading for big things.

But come the end of primary school, I went for a bunch of exams and asked my mum if I could just go to a 'normal school'; a school with more people like me. I missed my people, I missed being around people that looked like me, I missed not having to

> **From a very young age you learn to act, to code switch, to take the bass out of your voice and make yourself small.**

explain why my food smelt or looked funny, I missed not having to constantly defend my blackness. I am, however, grateful for the time I spent there as it taught me real early that this is life. This is the game, this is the chessboard of life and you must move the pieces strategically. All of this at such a young age? Why should you be thinking about that at 11 years old?

I switched school to a state secondary and then all the inner-city kids mocked me for how posh I was, and as time passed I evolved into this little hybrid kid who could talk to anyone regardless of the room.

After an hour-long sit down with Charlie, I got the nod. It was agreed that RDCWest would run on Mondays out of Paddington Recreation Ground, *but* under a few conditions. The most important condition was that I had to come to the main RDC session on Tuesdays to get a better understanding of the RDC culture, the nuances, the things that made RDC different. I agreed and that was that.

Committing to RDCWest on Mondays and RDC on Tuesdays was a big deal for me. It meant that I could no longer go to my Tuesday night track session with Dulwich Runners, or their weekly Wednesday night run. Ideally Wednesdays would now be my rest day after a punchy start to the running week.

RDCWest wasn't just run by myself; I did it in partnership with my dear friend Ellie Wood, who I had met while we were both based at Westminster. Our friendship grew over our love of running and raving and she worked for England Athletics, so it was the perfect fit.

On Monday nights RDCWest concentrated more on coached sessions where Ellie or I would lead a workout on the road. A lot of it was interval-type training where we would use our environment to guide the session, using steps, walls, benches, playgrounds and anything else we could find to spice up the session, adding plyometrics in workouts to help strengthen our bodies. We had smaller groups, wider roads and, due to our geographical location, it was easier for us to access big green spaces like Regent's Park, Hyde Park, Green Park and St James's Park, so our Monday session became the place that people would come to experiment with their bodies. For longer sessions we would take to the canal and do long reps of a kilometre, a mile or sometimes two. It was like track running but on the street. As we knew the area so well, we would take people to all the nooks and crannies of the city that only the locals get to see.

While our RDCWest Monday session was ticking along nicely, as promised I had started to attend the Tuesday night session at RDC. At first, I was very quiet and sat at the back of the room so I could see everything and everyone. I just wanted to get the lay of the land and see where I fitted in. Who were my people, my tribe, my new friends or – as we would later be referred to – my 'crew within the crew'?

From time to time, people would come in with medals from races that they had run, some as recently as the weekend before. They would attach letters or notes to the medals that Charlie would read in housekeeping.

Now let me set the scene for you: housekeeping was like church and my good friend and mentor Charlie was the pastor. It was both uplifting and emotional. Just imagine a room the size of a big class-room, with a stage at the front and tiered seats going up in levels so the people at the front are sat low and the people at the back are sat high up.

Charlie would say, 'As adults, when was the last time someone applauded you? Or just told you you are awesome at what you do or you're an amazing human being?' For most people it's not recent at all. It's something that I'd never really thought of. As kids you get congratulated all the time but as adults, unless you do something pretty epic, you won't find a room full of people applauding you.

Some of the notes would be short, a simple time and a 'great race' or 'terrible race' comment with the name attached. Others would write small novels explaining what happened, when and why it happened. Regardless of length, Charlie would read them out, then present each runner with their medal as if they were accepting Gold at the Olympics. Regardless of what the time or race was we would all stand and clap, shout, scream, cheer, bang tables, bang walls, anything and everything so that that person would feel loved and appreciated. It meant something, it felt special. *This* was community, *this* was togetherness.

I started to relax a little, and slowly but surely I started to feel more comfortable. I started talking to people from all walks of life, the kind of people that I had never met before – believe it or not, before meeting with Charlie I don't think I had been to Shoreditch on purpose. And I thought 1948 was a year not a place and I wasn't going to pretend that it was any other way. Just writing these words seems weird even now as I think to myself, how could I have never met someone that does this or that job? I'd never met a historian, a creative director of a marketing or ad company. I'd never met someone who was a videographer or photographer for real, a designer who'd designed some of the things that I was actually wearing. I'd never met anyone that worked in the office at Nike, someone with their own clothing label or someone who was looking for funding for their tech company. I knew nothing of this world that I was now knee-deep in. But that was the beauty of it. When we all walked through those doors and changed into our running kit we were stripped of our uniforms or clothing that made us identifiable.

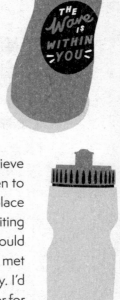

Now we were all just runners, just ourselves, a community from all walks of life *talking* and sharing their worlds.

t felt like I'd come home. I was surrounded by weirdos just like me, and I use that term 'weirdos' with all the love in my heart. When I say weirdos I mean people who just didn't seem like they fitted the mould of what society had told me was 'the norm'. But I guess my idea of the norm was very different to others. As time has passed my norm has definitely shifted, but at the time meeting unusual people like that was new and fresh. Being around all that love helped me realise that my love cup was still missing some sauce.

'What exactly is happening in Berlin? And when is the next one? I want in!'

Soon after I heard that a few people were going to Germany to run the Berlin half marathon, explore the city and party hard after. So, being the inquisitive, curious soul that I am, I started to ask questions. 'What exactly is happening in Berlin? And when is the next one? I want in!'

I found out that there was a thing called Bridge The Gap (BTG), founded by Mike Saes, Charlie Dark and Jessie Zapo. (Mike Saes also founded a crew called Bridge Runners and Jessie Zapo founded Girls Run NYC. Both out in New York.) The point of Bridge The Gap was to literally bridge the gap between running crews, meaning they could learn about each other in a bid to bring everyone closer together. Sharing worlds, sharing cultures, sharing loves for music, food, coffee, everything that made your crew different yet with so much in common.

Crews would either gather at a pre-existing race or create a race or experience of their own. If it was a race that already existed, like a 10k, half marathon or marathon, it was the host city crew's job to organise a weekend of events and activities that would showcase the city and its crew. Leaders would send the bat signal out inviting everyone and letting everyone know how to enter the race, or codes would be sent out for entry.

It was an opportunity to share local culture, art, routes, creativity and your passion with new friends from different places that realistically you'd never otherwise meet. The idea was that you'd see the city through the eyes of a local, not as a tourist. BTGs were breeding grounds for ideas and creativity, think tanks filled with people who were up for doing new and interesting things, and it was something that I'd never really been a part of before.

The main groups that I knew of in the beginning were RunDemCrew in London, England, Bridge Runners in New York, USA, Patta Running Club in Amsterdam, Netherlands, Paris Run Club in France, Harbour Runners in Hong Kong, AFE in Tokyo, Japan, NBRO in Copenhagen, Denmark and Graviteam in Berlin, Germany. And they all had to start somewhere.

Starting a running club or crew or organisation involves far more work than many people that I have spoken to think. Not just a running club, any kind of club. I just want to put that out there now. It's not something to start on a whim. If you want it to work you have to be committed and dedicated. Once you start, you can't just decide you don't want to do it anymore. Well, that's a lie, of course you can, you can do what you like. But people will be depending on you.

By setting up a club you're saying, *I promise that on this day at this time I or one of my representatives will be there for you and I or we won't let you down.* That's what people hear when you tell them to come to your club.

So, if you're thinking of starting a running club, the first thing that I would do if I were you is ask yourself honestly and genuinely, no nonsense, 'Why exactly is it that I want to start this club?' Make a list of the things that you want to accomplish. Are you starting the club

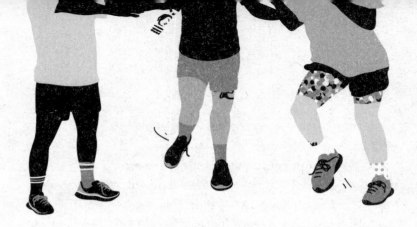

for yourself? Are you starting it for someone else? Are you starting it so you can run with your friends and other like-minded people? Do you see that there is something missing? Is it about representation of a particular group of people that you feel are currently underserved or not represented? Is it about community? Performance? Or both? Or are you doing it for clout? For kicks? Or the gram? For money, a brand deal or a career? Who do you want to come to your club? Is your club for everyone, or are you targeting a particular age group, demographic, sexuality or gender, geographical area or pace group? Do you want to see yourself in the group? Is it for you or for them? How often will you run? Where will you run? Where will you meet, start, finish? Will there be a bag drop? Who will help or support you?

It doesn't matter why you are doing it, as long as you are honest.

It doesn't matter why you are doing it, as long as you are honest and you can articulate what you are doing or want to do if asked, or when sharing your idea or enlisting others for your new group.

My advice to you is to think about these things, *but* try not to allow yourself to be overwhelmed. When our group TrackMafia started we had no answers to 99.9 per cent of those questions. All the three of us knew – me, Jeggi and Jules – was that we were friends who liked to run, we wanted to get used to running faster, we wanted to be more consistent. We would run on Thursdays at the Paddington Recreation

Ground track after work and in the beginning no one else was invited.

I am telling you all of this because I really want you to know what my running community means to me. I really want you to know how being part of different running communities has helped to mould me and my thinking. I have been part of, managed or set up groups that are driven by a number of different things from different types of communities: performance driven, brand driven, funding driven, charity or third sector driven, or simply numbers driven. This put me in a position that allowed me to see a lot more of what was happening in the running world than I ever thought I would. It showed me that many types of runs and clubs and people exist outside of what many deem the norm. It moulded my life and without it I would be very different. As a dear friend of mine said, 'Being in this space has accelerated your growth, morphed you into something that you never envisaged.'

y running community has opened doors for me and given me access to a world that quite simply I would never have dreamed of. If you said that I'd get to meet, let alone work with, the likes of Kevin Hart, Eliud Kipchoge, Michael Johnson, Tiger Woods, Alyson Felix, Paula Radcliffe or Mo Farah in real life I would have laughed at you and said, 'How? Under what circumstances would that happen? Please tell me as I don't see that in my future.' I remember standing on the side of the track in Monza, Italy, for Nike as Kipchoge attempted to break two hours for the marathon for the first time in history. Kevin Hart came over with a mic and camera crew and asked me to comment. I pretended like this was normal; meanwhile I'm thinking to myself, how the hell is this happening? I knew the answer. Running had brought me here and it was my job to make sure that others knew that this destination existed.

I understand and acknowledge that this is Cory's life, and that running may not have the same kind of impact on your life. I'm saying that you may never find out what you're capable of achieving if you don't take that first step followed by that first 'hello'.

Had you told me that because of running and my community I'd get to travel the world or have a dream job I would have said, 'How?' But more importantly, had you said that through my running community I would have been able to work with, inspire, mentor and be inspired and mentored by some amazing people – especially young people – I would have also said, 'How?' My running community has transported me to a place I never envisaged and empowered me to live my best life. So thank you to everyone involved.

I have said on countless occasions that running is boring, and I still think it's boring. *But* it's that commitment to sitting in the void, in that meditative state between boredom and monotony, where putting one foot in the front of the other becomes magical. Your

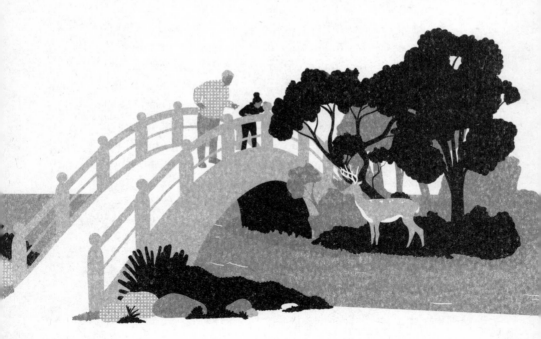

community can help you find that space, that place.

W hen I set out to run a group or crew or club, or simply an organisation, I said I wanted to accomplish five things that all seem to be rooted in access and community. To this day those five things have not changed:

1 I wanted to run in spaces in places where other people said you should not run;

2 I wanted to get more young people running;

3 more women and girls running;

4 more people of colour running; and

5 I wanted people to be less intimidated by speed and track, because it's not true that track is only for those that are fast – the track should be the place that you feel safe at, the place you go to play and experiment.

FINISH

Over the years I have witnessed people do some crazy and beautiful things either for the sake of the run or for the sake of the community of runners that you love. Many years ago I was in Copenhagen, Denmark, to run the Copenhagen Half Marathon. It was a race that frequently featured on our annual crew running calendar. Our friend and teammate was in another country on a stag do, dancing the night away. I phoned him and said, 'Dude, there are a few VIP race spaces knocking about for this half marathon tomorrow if you're up for it . . .' He booked a flight, left the club in the middle of the night, boarded a plane and I met him at the start line with his race pack. He ran the half marathon with us then partied a li'l more.

Charlie has always said that if you do not run you must cheer. And that is what this community does. People literally travel all over the world just to support their friends, and sometimes complete strangers. Many of us have driven through the night, gone without sleep or slept in ridiculous places or positions, just to be there, as we know that others have either done it for us or they would. That's what community does; it's there for you no matter what.

Many years ago, with a simple, 'You guys have a lot in common. You should talk,' Charlie introduced me to Ivo Gormley. Ivo is the founder of a charity called GoodGym. It's a community of people who get fit by doing good. A community who run and walk to help local community organisations and isolated older people by doing practical tasks. I ran the Hackney and Westminster branch of GoodGym for a few years and learnt that a run can be so much more than a run. A run can be about helping those that are less fortunate than yourself, or simply showing others that they can make a difference with their feet. That community has done some amazing things, and it still does. We would run to old people's homes and sing, we'd help to paint and decorate church halls or youth centres, build stone pizza ovens to help feed the homeless and others in need. Collect clothes for charities and hand them out. This is another side to the things that people will do for community, and it's such a beautiful

> **Charlie has always said that if you do not run you must cheer.**

thing.

And then of course, there's TrackMafia, the track baby that was born out of everything that I've mentioned above and a whole lot more. The craziest thing about TrackMafia's beginnings is it was started by three friends who just wanted to run together. I met Jules at RDCWest, Jeggi at RDC. We all bonded over our mutual cynicism, love of good coffee, good food and of course running.

In the beginning, that was it. And to be honest even after all the beautiful gifts that running has given us, that reason has remained the same. To run together and share space and time. What shall we do? We used to say: Break Bread and Share Miles. In any order, anytime, anywhere, even all at the same time. TrackMafia started because the three of us missed going to track sessions that we all couldn't attend for one reason or other. So while we were in my office we all decided that we'd run on Thursdays. We'd try some workouts that we'd been researching. We wanted to do what the greatest runners in the world were doing, so we started looking up workouts that Ethiopian and Kenyan runners used. We looked at what other great coaches were doing around the world, what workouts they were giving their athletes, what our favourite athletes Tirunesh Dibaba and Genzebe Dibaba in Ethiopia were doing. Then we tapped into our running community. Who else was doing things a little differently, not just with running but with intervals, track, speed workouts and community? We started speaking to Knox from New York who was a Nike coach and founded the New York crew, The Black Roses. We asked him what kind of workouts he was doing and what he was doing with his groups. We had

FaceTimes, phone calls, email chains, texts, WhatsApp, every kind of communication as we really wanted to get it right for OUR BODIES.

A few years after TrackMafia was born I started as the London Head Coach for the Nike Run Club. Big thank you to Nike for seeing something in me that I hadn't seen myself yet. Nike had run clubs based at stores and other locations all over the world. I was invited over to New York for training and to meet the Global Head Coach, Coach Bennett, and all my coachly colleagues from, guess where? *All over the world.* This was another community that I was introduced to. On the trip I may have met all the coaches, but through Nike and an app and Instagram and other social media platforms I had access to thousands of people who were running just like me. Then when I moved to LA and joined Apple Fitness+ my community got even bigger and expanded beyond running into an even broader fitness and wellness community giving me even more inspiration. And YOU

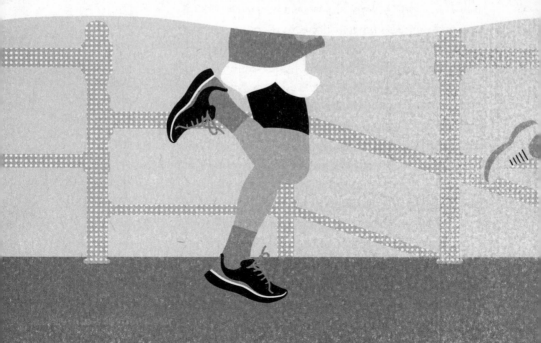

TOO have access to these apps and other apps where you get to meet like-minded people. People with similar goals to you. Not just running goals but life goals. And the beauty of these fitness apps is some of them actually have real-life running meets set up, so you can meet and run with people in a safe environment. That's a great place to mingle with others and suggest meeting outside of the group for your own little 'Crew within the Crew' runs.

All in all there's a lot out there. I know at times it might be daunting. But I can promise you if you commit to finding your community, or starting your own, you'll learn a lot about running and a lot more about people and, if you're lucky, what it really means to be family. Like all things, you might not get it right or find the right folks the first time. It doesn't mean they don't exist, it just means you haven't found them yet. *And* it's not a strike or misstep, mishap or miscalculation, it's something else you get to tick off the list of done that and learnt this.

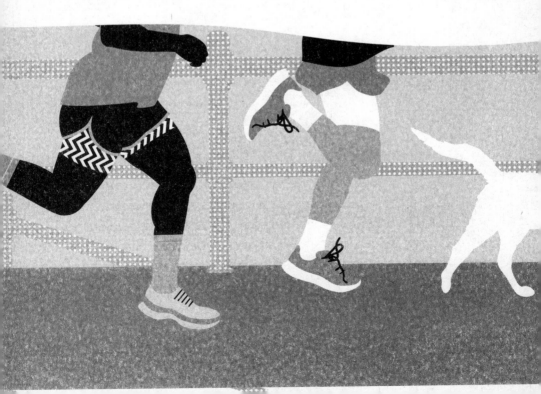

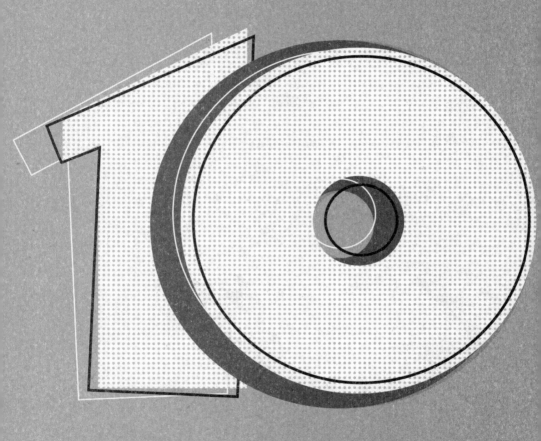

All You Need Is Need Is Rhythm & Grit

When I laced up my shoes for the first time as the self-proclaimed fat kid who loves cake, I never thought at any point I would write about it, let alone fill a whole book about this magical running journey of mine. It's a journey that has completely changed the course of my life, and in some part, the lives of others. They say that allowing your stream of consciousness to fill a page can help to release emotions and offer insight into the inner workings of your mind, meaning that just allowing whatever is in your head at that moment in time to pour out of your heart and head can do wonders for the soul. I have to say that for me, this was the most definitely the case.

As I scribbled in my little notebook and tapped away furiously on my keyboard it was as if I was reliving every moment, every run, the highs, the lows, the laughter and the tears. The races through the woods, through underground car parks and shopping malls, on top of mountains, along beaches. Solo running, relays, running with friends, chanting for others and willing them on . . . People screaming my name as I trundled on through cheer zones in different countries and cities. Broken records, missed PBs, headaches and heartache — the list is endless.

All the things that have come together to put this BIG SMILE on my face – *so many memories* that all lead back to one thing – THE RUN.

Back then, I wasn't always smiling, and when I was that smile wasn't as wide or as bright. I think back to a world without running, a world where I physically didn't have the ability to move freely. Back to a time when I didn't have faith or trust in myself or my body. A time when I had no clue what I was doing with my life, where I wanted to go or what I wanted to do. I just seemed to exist, floating from job to job, hobby to hobby, searching for something, but not quite sure what. It's like when you're hungry, but have no idea what you want to eat, you just head to the fridge in search of something that might fill a hole. That was my life before finding my INSPIRATION, my true purpose.

The more I thought about this the more I realised that the moment I really, really started to run physically, I stopped running mentally. I stopped hiding from myself and in turn stopped hiding much of my true self from others. And that Cardio Confidence slowly started to chip away at my guarded world. That Cardio Confidence gave me purpose and offered me clarity in a world that for a long time had felt hazy. It is a by-product of no longer being afraid to be vulnerable and alone with my thoughts, of hours and hours of pounding the pavement come rain, hail, sleet or snow. That Cardio Confidence is what came from committing to hours of self-reflection and literally blood, sweat and tears.

That's the thing about this running thing; if you let it, I honestly believe that it genuinely has the power to change your world. And for it to change your world, you don't have to be special, or gifted. You don't have to have started running when you were a child. You can start now, TODAY or tomorrow. And in the beginning, all you need is you, some kicks and what is already waiting for you right outside your door.

I look at my life, my world, and ask myself this question. What in my life don't I owe to running? I look around and everything is because of running; I met Jules, my wife, through running, it's given me the opportunity to travel the world, meet the most amazing people and see their cities through their eyes, not the eyes of a tourist. All these people have become friends.

My job came out of running. Therefore everything I own, all the places that I visit, the food I eat, the gifts I buy, my HEALTH and HAPPINESS, is in some way connected to running.

I know starting out can be daunting, but as I said trust in yourself, trust in the process and trust that the road will give you what you need. I didn't say you would like what the road gives you or that you will love it, because in the beginning you probably won't. But like many things in life, it begins with the first step. It begins with starting slowly and not being judgemental or comparing yourself with others. Of course, there may be tears, injuries, setbacks. *But* that is why, in my humble opinion, running is one of the greatest metaphors for LIFE.

I wrote this book as a love letter to running and my old self in the hope that it would speak to you, perhaps help you find a piece of yourself that you may have lost, misplaced or not even known existed. I wrote this book so you could learn from my mistakes, so that you either didn't make the same ones or at least knew where the path might lead. I wrote this book as I want YOU to use it like a little cheat sheet. I want you to come back to it as and when you need to.

I know that at times it can feel like it's just you, like no one is there to cheer for you, to will you on, to scream your name and tell you that you're doing it. To tell you that you're worthy. To tell you that the one thing that you can control is YOU.

Running has the ability to change you and those around you, the way that you see the world and the world sees you. *But*, in order for this to happen, you have to let running in. KNOCK KNOCK.

Acknowledgements

Lyn – Thank you for being my biggest cheerleader, for raising me, loving me, guiding me and helping me understand that there was no rush . . . you believed that I would find my way, and because you did, I DID. Thank you for teaching me that you must share what you have regardless of how much or how little you have. Thank you for teaching me that to go forward, at times you must go back. Thank you for teaching me that what will be will be.

Janeen – Thank you for always being there to support me and make me feel like I was enough, that you were proud of me. Quietly gassssssing me up. ☺

Julia Good – To my Jules, to the one I love, to my partner in crime, my CO-D, collaborator and creator. To the one who has sacrificed so much to help build what we have. You've been right by my side every step of the way, listening to me, pushing me, loving me, believing in me. To the one who understands me and somehow manages to continue to decipher the Beefy code. Thank you for being you and letting me be me. I love you.

Dean Forbes and Nic Taylor – I hear that in this life all you need is two good friends to not just survive, but thrive. You have been just that for over thirty years now and without you, my brothers, I wouldn't have made it this far, so thank you for the inspiration and constant counsel. DON'T CHANGE my friends . . . DON'T CHANGE.

Eugene Minogue – Thank you for everything, dude. I strolled into a community space with a silly idea and you gave me your mentorship, your friendship and a career. Thank you for treating me like family and helping to change my life, my friend.

Patrica Fairclough OBE – I owe so much to you, if only you knew. You took me aside and spoke to me, just like how my gran, mother or aunt would. The talking-to that you gave me will forever be part of, not just my coaching style, but me.

Sam Bell – Thank you for introducing me to the gift that keeps on giving. Thank you for all the support and, most importantly, thank you for not laughing when I said that the marathon life was for me.

Dulwich Runners – Thank you for taking a beginner runner under your wing and teaching him all about a world he knew nothing about. Thank you for inspiring me to try harder and for being honest with me about what I needed to do to take my running and my life to the next level.

Charlie Dark MBE – Nothing I write here will do justice to what you have done for me, my friend. You have been a role model to me and so many others. You have taught me so much about myself and what it takes to be part of change, part of something that is far more important than myself. You showed me a world that I didn't even know existed and proceeded to help guide me through it. Thank you for showing me where the ladder was and NOT PULLING IT UP. You taught us all that there's space for everyone.

Babs (Barbara Brunner) – Thank you for everything that you have done for me, you're an amazing human being who I love and care for very much. Thank you for what you've taught me about myself and my body, for the number of times I have gone to you broken and said – Please fix me! How long will it take? – and you've said we can do it but it's going to hurt. Thanks for helping to teach me that I am in control and can do anything I put my mind to.

Jeggi – You believed in a team before one even existed and without that belief, there would be no us. So, thank you, my brother, thank you for believing that there was space to be made for what we were bringing to the table. DISRUPTION! Lol.

Tom – Thank you for believing in the wave, my friend, even when we had nothing to ride it. Luckily, we know a few people who 'know what they're doing!' 😊

TrackMafia – Thank you for believing in building something that helped others see what it meant to be a team.

Mike Saes and Cedric Hernandez (Bridge Runners) – You truly made New York feel like my second home and helped me understand the true beauty of Bridge the Gap, the global running community that you helped create amidst the chaos.

RunDemCrew and Bridge the Gap Community – All of you helped me relive my twenties in my thirties, and taught me so much about the power of community and what happens when like-minded people all over the world come together with peace and love in their hearts. Thanks for showing me your city and sharing your world, a world that helped give me a new lease on life.

Black Roses and Patta Running Team – Thank you for being committed to these words, 'Let's Build'.

WRU Crew – Thank you for sharing your world with me, one run at a time, solidifying my belief that regardless of where you are, if you're with your people, you're home.

Chop – Thank you for being my friend and collaborator, for believing in me, for challenging me creatively and pushing me, for teaching me more than I knew I needed to learn. Thank you for always being there whether in person, on a call, email or text. Thank you for taking the time to share your world and your knowledge with someone, when you didn't have to.

Rory Fraser – Thank you for spreading the good word, my friend, and you know exactly what I'm talking about. 😊

Ruth Hooper – It was you who gave me my first opportunity at Nike; I remember our conversation like it was yesterday. You said trust in yourself and your own ability and it won't take long for you to get where you want to go. So, I trusted you, the brand and the process.

Fodz (Foday Dumbaya) – There is much to thank you for, my brother, but right here, right now, I want to thank you for all the early morning meets where we would just sit and break bread, no agenda, no plan, just talk of positivity, progression and means and ways of breaking barriers and bringing our people with us on this wild rollercoaster ride.

Harry Jameson – Thank you for talking me into taking a chance.

Francesca, Carly and Cindy – Thank you for helping me write the book my younger self needed to read.

YOU – I have said this since the first event I ever put on. I didn't do it alone . . . and still don't. Without you, the people, without my community, my friends and the friends that I haven't made yet, I'd be all alone standing in a void screaming, shouting and running alone. So, thank you for trusting in me, believing me and, more importantly, giving me the time and space to grow and keep growing. A lot happened before I arrived here, BUT you helped to create this . . . SO, THANK YOU!

Info & Inspo

Crew culture

These are some of the running crews that inspire me and remind me that there's more to this running thing than just running. It's about community and it's always good to have people around you that inspire you, especially people who look like you, people who make you feel seen, people who understand what it's like.

London

@**Run.Dem.Crew** www.rundemcrew.com
@**TrackMafia_** www.trackmafia.co.uk
@**FlyGirlCollective** flygirlcollective.co
@**UltraBlackRunning**

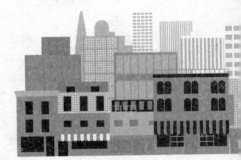

New York

@**BridgeRunners**
@**WRUCrew** werunuptown.com
@**GirlsRunNYC**
@**OldManRunClub**
@**HarlemRun**
@**BlackRosesNYC** www.blackrosesnyc.com

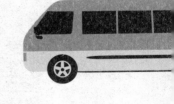

Los Angeles

@**GoodVibes_tc**
@**KeepItRunHundred**
@**KoreaTownRunClub**
@**BlackRosesNYC** www.blackrosesnyc.com

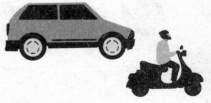

Elsewhere

@DistrictRunningCollective www.districtrunningcollective.com
– Washington DC
@PattaRunningTeam www.patta.nl/pages/patta-running-team
– Amsterdam and Rotterdam
@BerlinBraves – Berlin
@harbourrunners – Hong Kong
@afe_tokyo – Tokyo
@prrc1936 – Seoul

Running culture

Long Distance longdistance.world
Born during the pandemic, a collection of stories and photographs told by and taken from runners across the world.

Tempo Journal tempojournal.com
A publication about the people who dedicate their lives, day by day and week by week, to the unglamorous sport of running.

Runner's World www.runnersworld.com/uk/, www.runnersworld.com
A globally circulated monthly magazine for runners of all skill sets. Great for learning about all things running. Where I went to for advice when I first started running. It's also home to my column 'Rhythm & Grit' and a place you can go to to find and enter races.

Athletics Weekly athleticsweekly.com
A monthly track and field magazine that covers news, results, fixtures, coaching and product advice for all aspects of track and field, cross-country, road racing and race walking.

FloTrack www.flotrack.org
Great for if you want to dig into everything track and field, with behind-the-scenes coverage.

Citius Mag citiusmag.com
Home to original running, track and field news, analysis, videos, newsletters, podcasts and humour.

Trail Running Mag www.trailrunningmag.co.uk
A magazine that covers the places, events, gear, fitness and training for all things related to trail running.

Women's Running UK www.womensrunning.com
Women's Running reports on training, nutrition and news to inspire female athletes to embrace their journey through running and beyond.

Men's Running UK mensrunninguk.co.uk
A running magazine for men featuring regular training plans, features and gear reviews for runners of all abilities.

Find a Race findarace.com
Great place to find a race to run.

parkrun www.parkrun.com
Free timed 5ks on Saturday morning all over the UK and parts of the USA.

England Athletics www.englandathletics.org
The governing body for the sport of athletics in England. It offers membership and is the development body for grassroots athletics and running clubs in England. It's great for finding clubs and qualifications.

British Athletics www.britishathletics.org.uk
The UK national governing body for the sport of athletics. Responsible for a number of high-level functions, including the provision of world-class performance athletics such as Great Britain and Northern Ireland international teams, rules and regulations for UK.

Lifestyle, Fitness 'n' Culture

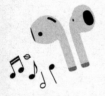

The following are great for tips and tricks on all things fitness-related that can help with running, from talk on nutrition to advice on sleep and playlists:

Men's Health www.menshealth.com
Women's Health www.womenshealthmag.com
Men's Fitness mensfitness.co.uk

I have always found the websites below very insightful as they all offer a window into fitness, running and the lifestyle that surrounds it through a different lens. Of course the running part of running is important, but so is everything else.

Esquire www.esquire.com
GQ www.gq.com
Men's Journal www.mensjournal.com
Refinery www.refinery29.com/en-us/running

Gear Patrol www.gearpatrol.com
A great resource for reviews on kit and tech you can use to help enhance your running experience.

Tom's Guide www.tomsguide.com
A great resource for reviews and tech you can use to help enhance your running experience as well as information on workouts.

Nutrition

Both of the experts below offer great advice on nutrition for life and for sport. They are also great at myth busting and telling you the truth about food:

Graeme Tomlinson **@thefitnesschef** www.fitnesschef.uk
Dr Hazel Wallace **@thefoodmedic** www.thefoodmedic.co.uk

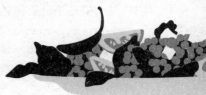

Apps

Apple Fitness+ www.apple.com/apple-fitness-plus/
Find yours truly on this app, either smiling and sweating in the background or talking in your ear, guiding or coaching you on a run in a Time To Run location somewhere in the world. Everyone is invited to the party and the community. Get access to thousands of video and audio workouts led by my awesome teammates – everything from HIIT to running to yoga. And guided meditations. Take it further with personalised metrics from Apple Watch. Find it in the Fitness app on iPhone, iPad, or Apple TV.

Nike Run Club apps.apple.com/gb/app/
nike-run-club-running-coach/id387771637
From expert coaches to an incredible community, the NRC running app has what you need to start running, keep running, and enjoy running more. Guided runs, training plans, pace tracker, running log, GPS distance tracker and more await. You might even find me coaching you on some of the guided runs.

Nike Training Club apps.apple.com/gb/app/
nike-training-club-fitness/id301521403
Gain tips for complete wellness with home workouts and healthy recipes that strengthen both the mind and body. Programmes are led by Nike Trainers, world-class personal trainers and wellness experts.

Strava apps.apple.com/gb/app/strava-run-ride-hike/
id426826309
Great for tracking data and finding like-minded people, communities and challenges. Useful if you start to dip your foot into other sports.

My Fitness Pal apps.apple.com/gb/app/
myfitnesspal-calorie-counter/id341232718
This is the app I used to track my daily calorie intake.

FootPath apps.apple.com/gb/app/footpath-route-planner/
id634845718
I find this app useful when you just want to draw a running route with your finger, and you want to check that you're on track.

All Trails apps.apple.com/gb/app/alltrails-hike-run-walk/
id405075943
Good app for finding easy hikes or trails nearby for running, cycling, walking or hiking.

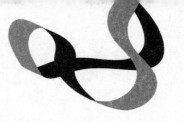
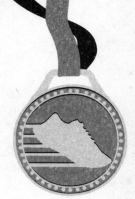

Giving back

I have worked with or for the following organisations, who all do their bit to uplift communities through, fitness, education and or food:

@TrapFruitsLondon trapfruitslondon.com
Encouraging healthy eating in the Black community and beyond.

@Badu_Sports www.thebaduway.com
BADU offers support to families, schools and local organisations through mentorship, running and sport. BADU's goal is to bridge the gap between what society has predetermined and what individuals, families and community are truly capable of achieving.

@GoodGym www.goodgym.org
GoodGym helps you get fit by doing good. They are a group of runners, walkers and cyclists who combine regular exercise with helping communities and by visiting elderly people and those in need.

@ForbesFamilyGroup forbesfamilygroup.com
A committed group offering to support initiatives and create opportunities at a grass-roots level through charity, not for profit and development programmes for Black and brown people. How can you turn your running hobby or club into more than a hobby?

@GirlsGottaRun www.girlsgottarun.org
My first trip to Ethiopia was to train at altitude and to work with Girls Gotta Run, who utilise running as a foundation for girls in Ethiopia to develop personal agency, community and mentorship.

@guapmag guap.co, instagram.com/guapmag

A youth-led new media platform dedicated to discovering, show-casing and nurturing emerging and under-represented creatives and communities. Guap have done a lot of work to highlight the benefits of running, wellness and the impact that it can have on your mental health and creativity.

Books

Here are the first three books on running I read:

Haruki Murakami, *What I Talk About When I Talk About Running* (Vintage, 2009) – Probably the very first running book I read. It speaks to running being a driving force as well as an escape. At the time I don't think I fully understood what he was talking about. I just thought it was beautiful writing and wished to one day be able to express my feelings on running the way he had.

Dean Karnazes, *Ultra Marathon Man: Confessions of an All Night Runner* (Penguin, 2006) – It honestly blew my mind that this dude pushed his body so far that he fell asleep when he was running. That made me feel like if he could do that, I could run to the bottom of the road. I could give up a few minutes a day to work on myself.

Christopher McDougall, *Born To Run: A Hidden Tribe, Super Athletes, and the Greatest Race the World Has Never Seen* (Profile, 2009) – This was the book that made me realise there was far more to running than I could ever have imagined. It was like a movie – secret tribes, superhuman athletes, a virtually unknown long-distance race and natural born heroes.

And here are some others I found equally inspiring:

Ed Caesar, *Two Hours: The Quest to Run the Impossible Marathon* (Penguin, 2016) – A book that captures the lives, training routines, the triumph and pain that comes with missed opportunities, and the proud ancestry of the amazing runners trying to make history and break 2 hours for a marathon.

Alison Mariella Désir, *Running While Black: Finding Freedom in a Sport That Wasn't Built for Us* (Portfolio, 2022) – A great book exploring the history of running, the reality of racism and racial restrictions in America, and the transformative power of running and its positive effects on people's mental health.

Mo Farah, *Twin Ambitions* (Hodder, 2016) – A personal account of the amazing life of Mo Farah. From humble beginnings to world-class athlete, and everything in between. A testament to hard work.

Adharanand Finn, *Running with the Kenyans* (Faber, 2013) – Adharanand ventures to Kenya to uncover the secrets of the fastest people on earth. It's books like these that make me fall in love with running even more. They live and breathe it every day.

Alexandra Heminsley, *Running Like a Girl: Notes on Learning to Run* (Windmill, 2014) – The inspiring, hilarious memoir of a 'Bridget Jones-like writer' (Washington Post) who transforms her life by learning to run. She had hopes of a blissful runner's high and immediate physical transformation but found instead miserable defeat before complete victory.

Scott Jurek, *Eat and Run* (Bloomsbury, 2013) – Great book about ultra runner Scott Jurek, showing the power of dedication and the important role food plays in your life as a runner.

Lopez Lomong, *Running for My Life: One Lost Boy's Journey from the Killing Fields of Sudan to the Olympic Games* (Thomas Nelson, 2012) – An incredible story about a world-class runner and his journey from being kidnapped by rebel soldiers in Sudan to becoming an Olympian for the USA.

Index

Page numbers in italics refer to illustrations